That Hair Thing

And The Sisterlocks Approach

JoAnne Cornwell

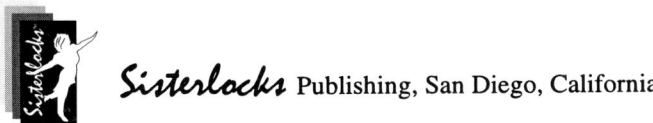

Sisterlocks Publishing, San Diego, California

That Hair Thing
And The Sisterlocks Approach

By
JoAnne Cornwell

Published by:
Sisterlocks Publishing
5663 Balboa Avenue, #355
San Diego, CA 92111

Internet: www.sisterlocks.com

All Rights Reserved. No part of this book may be reproduced or transmitted in any form or by any means, electronic or mechanical, including photocopying, recording or by any information storage and retrieval system without written permission from the author, except for the inclusion of brief quotations .

Library of Congress Catalog Card Number: 97-91747

ISBN 0-9657426-5-2 (pbk.)

Copyright 1997 by JoAnne Cornwell
First Printing 1997
Printed in the United States of America

Dedication:

This work is dedicated to my mother, Dora Lee Smith Jenkins who, now in spirit, is my greatest inspiration.

4   That Hair Thing

I'd be willing to bet though, that a poll of first impressions of those reading these lines would produce very nearly the same set of assumptions about our dear gentleman as I have just proposed. How can I be so sure of this? Well, I'm betting that those who would pick up and read a book like this one, share in common many of the same symbolic message systems as I do. To the extent this is true, I'm betting that they have learned to respond in similar ways as I have to certain dress codes.

Hair is another one of the many important symbolic systems we use to give our lives meaning. Some would say that hair codes are just as superficial as they believe dress codes to be. From my perspective though, both are deeply connected to our sense of who we think we are, both on an interpersonal level, and in the ways we relate to others. Hair, like other systems, does not get its meaning from just anywhere. Its meaning depends on the relationship it has to, and the reinforcement it gets from the systems coming into play in our daily living.

I've already mentioned a couple of these systems. It's fairly easy to come up with a dozen or so ways we typically use to communicate non-verbally, who we think we are. These might include our style of speech, facial and hand gestures, style of body movement, responses to authority and our reactions to age, gender, race and social class. In with these go the ways we adorn ourselves and yes, the ways we wear our hair.

With this in mind, let's go one step further. When the majority of the message systems in our lives support one another, our existence feels both normal and natural. In fact, the many systems of meaning in a person's life can reinforce one another quite seamlessly. When this happens, the **truth value** of the messages sent and received from those around us, goes up. What this means is that these systems are not seen as 'Symbolic' at all. They are simply seen as 'True'. If someone's culture is doing the job it's supposed to do - that is to say, the job that human cultures have sought to accomplish up to this day - the person

---

Hair is another one of the many important symbolic systems we use to give our lives meaning.

will end up believing that their reality is the primary one. It becomes simply REALITY to them.

The question for African Americans becomes, "Is our culture doing the job it's supposed to do?" Of course, there is not one answer for all African Americans, but consider this: Ordinarily, when people find themselves fully enveloped in the symbolic systems of their culture, they tend not even to be aware that their way of life is just one of many 'normal' ways of living that vary from one perspective to another. They do not tend to view their existence in terms of any other possible ways of existing; no other way may have been thought of, seen or explored. These people are not generally aware of the factors that make their approach to life unique and distinct from others (i.e. class, race, etc.).

If you were to ask this type of person, "What are you?" they might very well volunteer, "Just a person," or perhaps, "Just an American." What else would they be? This is often the response I hear from European American students and individuals in the corporate world who are members of the majority culture. Those of us who know people like this also know that they can be quite maddening to deal with if they are in positions of power and concepts of diversity are not part of their primary reality.

What I am saying here is that messages become truer, or even larger than life, when they are a part of (symbolic) systems that support each other. Messages become less true, or weaker on the other hand, where the support of other systems is missing.

Many African Americans, for example, lead lives where messages conveyed by speech, gestures, dress, language or racial characteristics work in conflict with one another. (i.e. My speech conveys one kind of message, but my physical appearance conveys another.) When this is the case, the strength (or truth value) of whatever statement is being made, invariably weakens. Living in this way can be extremely confusing and stressful, especially when this occurs during our formative years when we are not aware of how symbolic message systems work or know how to strengthen them. Here is an example to illustrate what I mean.

Envision the following scenario: Mother spends an extra amount of time one morning preparing her 10 year old for school because on this particular day, the girl will be bussed to a school across town. The doting mother adds extra barrettes to her daughter's neatly braided plaits or 'puff balls', does not skimp on the Vaseline, and chooses the brightest colors in which to adorn her precious child. Need I say more? By three o'clock, our daughter has learned that the stuff on her head is not exactly hair, that she is greasy and that she has no sense of style. How many of us experienced this in one way or another when we were children? Uninformed, insensitive comments and actions may not even be intentional. They may simply be the reflection of a different set of codes. Their effect however, is still damaging.

Tension is always created when the symbolic message systems in a person's life come into conflict with others that are coded and understood differently. Once the little girl in our example leaves the home setting where her systems may operate supportively, she may find herself assaulted by opposing systems that process and evaluate her ways differently. How many of us, when we were little, thought we were just children in the world, until some incident - usually racial - told us otherwise! Many times, this kind of brutalizing message is conveyed without ever using the language of speech at all.

Like it or not, most of us are not able to simply ignore the systems that pass negative judgment on us. While our 10 year old may value and love the care and affirmation she receives at home, this may not be enough to diminish the sheer weight of the opposing judgments against her. At the very least, she will experience some confusion over the situation, and if she has a healthy ego, it will also make her angry! Despite this, she will probably internalize some feelings of guilt or embarrassment, especially if she feels forced to conform to these

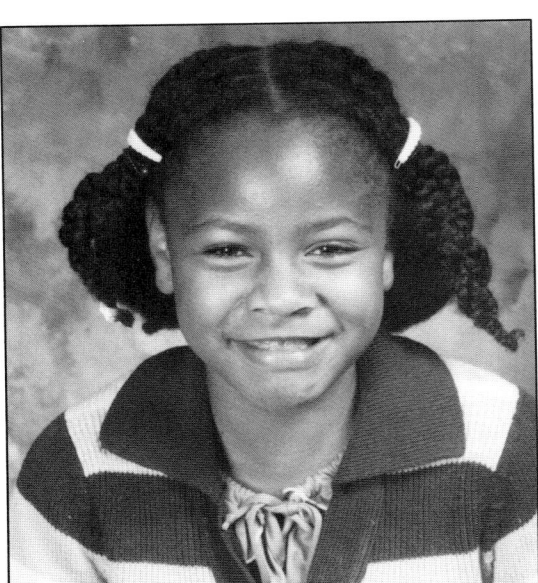

other systems.

By the time we reach adulthood, most African Americans I am aware of have developed a sixth sense about the symbolic systems that activate our lives. We know very well that there are powerful codes at work that seek to negate or diminish our own, because we have seen the value of our ways routinely called into question for most of our lives. Many of us for example, may "dress for success" from 9 to 5, but enjoy looking, feeling and acting more ethnic after hours and on weekends. Or, we may speak standard English when answering the company phone, but talk that other talk with intimate friends and family. Though it may not be absolutely necessary to abandon the systems in our lives that first served to give it meaning, we are mindful that their meaning will be under-valued by the majority culture.

Unlike in the earlier example I gave, where someone can be totally unaware that other systems exist, most African Americans I know feel constant pressure from external messages, that must be resisted in order to maintain a healthy balance in their lives. This makes us acutely, sometimes painfully aware that certain of our ways are precisely 'other than' what is supposed to be 'normal.' Through this experience we come to understand how things like history, class, race and other factors can affect how we develop a sense of who we are. When asked, "What are you?," we will rarely self-identify as 'just a person,' 'just an American,' 'just a woman' or for that matter, just-an-anything. This tends to be true of African Americans and others whose race or ethnicity is central to their sense of who they are.

When it comes to our physical characteristics like skin color and hair, we often come up against conflicting messages. Our appearance may be <u>saying</u> one thing (we think...) but it may <u>mean</u> quite another, depending on where we are or who we are with at any given moment. When this happens, is our own hair reality a primary reality for us? That is to say, do we feel that our own hair type is normal and natural?

For the same reason that African American women do not tend to think of ourselves as 'just women' or 'just Americans,' we also do not tend to think of our hair as 'just hair.' This is not news to anyone born female and black in this country. Our hair is felt to be something other than what is

The Symbolism Of Our Hair

When it comes to our physical characteristics like skin color and hair, we often come up against conflicting messages. Our appearance may be saying one thing (we think...) but it may mean quite another

considered normal and natural - Caucasian-type hair. How does this play out for us? What are the reasons why our hair symbolism carries such a powerfully negative message for us? What keeps our culture from doing its job when it comes to our hair?

Let's look first at hair symbolism for Americans in general. I've noticed that the symbolism of hair is expressed primarily in terms of three features; **styling, color** and **length**. It is possible to get a feel for someone's self perception, age, class status and even politics from the symbolism of these three features of their hair. No attribute of hair is ever 'value free', though this may seem to be the case at times. Instead, every attribute sets off value judgments of one kind or another, and the astute wearer can use combinations of attributes to send messages that will work to their advantage.

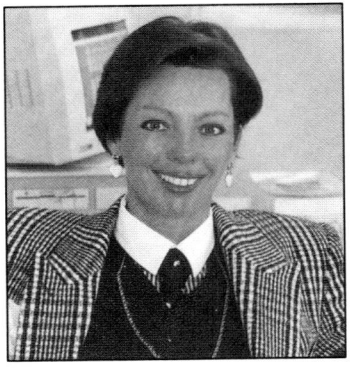

For instance, some combinations of length, color and style can be used to send messages that increase the wearer's chances for employment. This might be seen in a short to moderate length, or a conservative color and style. Some attributes may make the wearer more acceptable as a public figure. In this category there are instances when graying hair is desirable. Other combinations of attributes send messages that say the wearer bears allegiance to a particular regional group, occupation or popular sub-culture.

Notice so far that the way I've been discussing hair here does not address the most important thing of all for <u>African-type</u> hair. That is, TEXTURE. You may

32   That Hair Thing

also notice in your daily life a similar kind of 'silent treatment' with regard to our natural hair texture. People rarely talk about this openly, as though it were our nasty little secret. The silence that surrounds this topic however, is really a kind of 'erasure.' It allows people to behave as though <u>all</u>

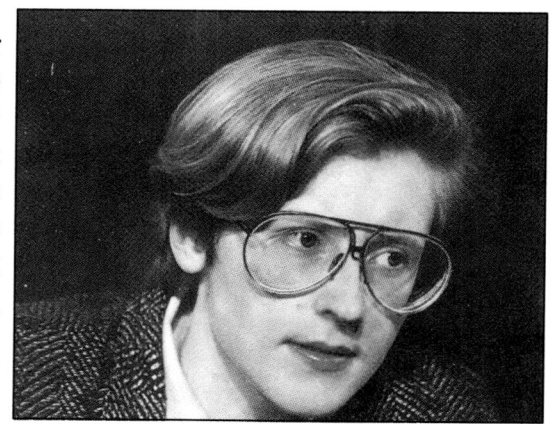

What hair-symbolism is at work here? What do the <u>length,</u> <u>color</u> and <u>styling of</u> the hair suggest to you about these individuals?

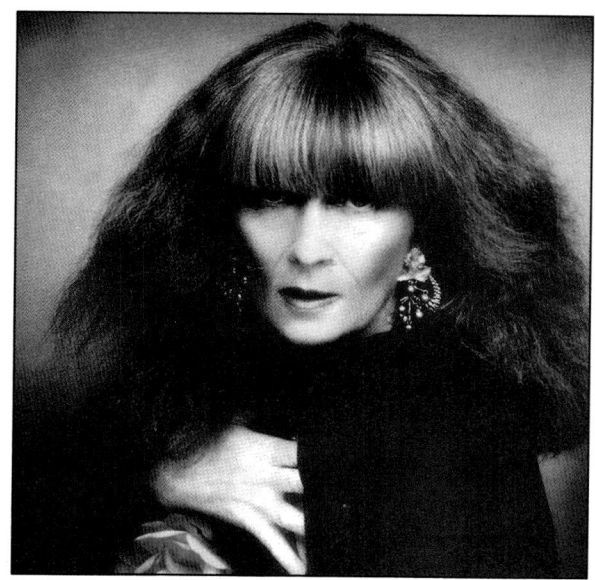

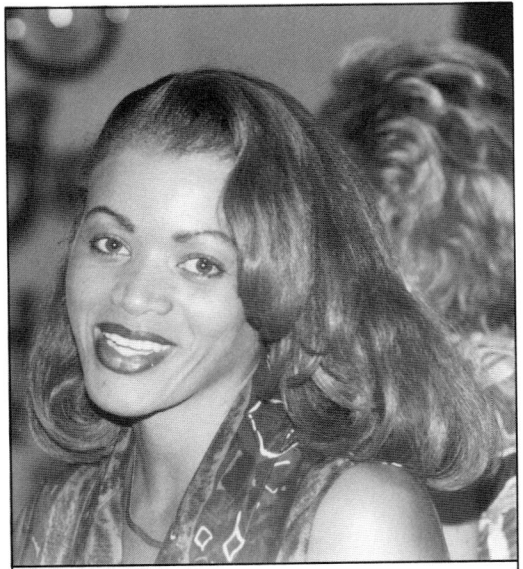

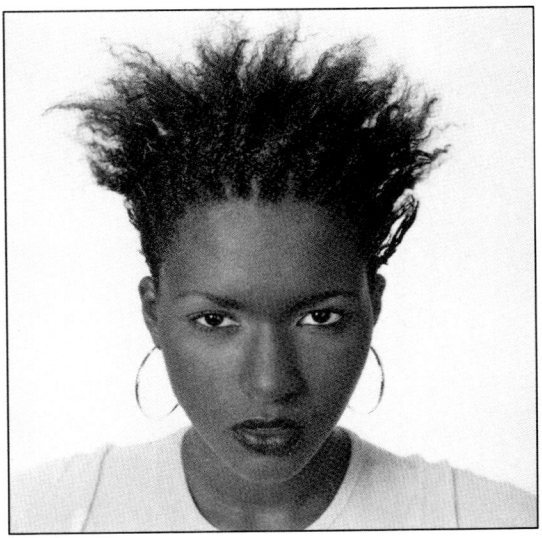

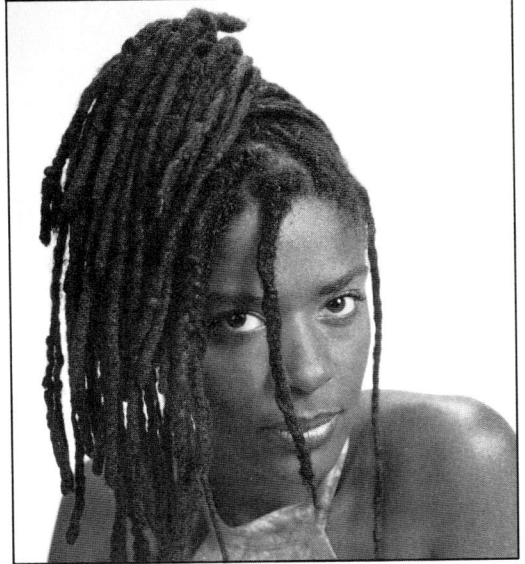

*Now, what hair-symbolism is at work here? Is is possible to consider **length, color** and **styling** of the hair alone, without also considering **texture**?*

hair types respond in the same ways as Caucasian hair types, and that **length,** **color** and **styling** remain the most significant features. Our issues however - those relating specifically to the hair's TEXTURE - are simply not part of the discussion, as if these issues did not exist.

In fact, the professional hair care industry is still very much in the habit of erasing texture from African-type hair in order for it to be considered suitable for standard hair styling procedures. In most beauty colleges, the <u>Standard Textbook of Cosmetology</u> is required reading for those becoming licensed to practice hair care. This text quite craftly promotes chemical relaxing as the norm.

*"**Chemical hair relaxing is the process of permanently rearranging the basic structure of <u>overly-curly</u> (!) hair into a straight form. When done professionally, it leaves the hair straight and in a <u>satisfactory</u> condition, to be set into <u>almost</u> any style.*"[1] (My emphasis)

What I am saying here is that texture for us makes ALL the difference. Are you aware of the deep symbolic message that texture sends in American culture (and in Western culture in general)? You may guess that it is primarily negative, but do you know why? Let me offer one explanation: 'Coily' hair structures in the human gene pool trace back to what is called the "Negroid substratum." To be blunt, this means that the more textured your hair is, the more closely it, and you, are associated with 'blackness.' Simply put, texture in hair sends a very strong racial message.

As most of us know, the idea of natural, racial hierarchy among human cultures was at the very core of thinking in Western civilizations for several centuries. In this way of thinking, black skin and attributes associated with African-type peoples (i.e. hair type, facial features, body proportions) were placed at the opposite lower extreme from white skin and certain other Caucasion attributes. The physical characteristics of African peoples were taken as symbols of biological inferiority, intellectual backwardness, and by extension, cultural degradation. Since blackness was defined as the **negation** of things like quality, intelligence and value, the negative content of the texture message was clear. This negative symbolic meaning remains with us today. It is what makes our hair something other than what is presumed to be normal and natural, and of course, desirable in this culture.

Because our way of thinking today is still embedded in this mentality, coily hair texture continues to set itself apart from the other attributes - **styling, color** and **length.** (Incidentally, coily hair textures are common to some Caucasian groups too, though this is seldom openly discussed.) We might sum things up in this way: Hair issues for African Americans are complicated because hair symbolism in this country is complicated. It is not only related to things like fashion, occupations and fad. Hair symbolism also relates to the politics of race.

The following example is intended to show how our hair issues have been surrounded in silence, and how this erasure sends a very powerful, negative message. Consider the following take-off on a seemingly harmless, tried-and-true approach to pitching hair care products in this country. You have heard this many times before: A stereotypical 'Buffy' sits in front of her mirror looking very plain. "How will I wear my hair?," she asks. After choosing miracle product-X, she is now glamorous, and ready for her night out with 'Tad.' Glimmering symbols of softness and femininity send the loud-and-clear message that miracle product-X will transform YOU TOO!

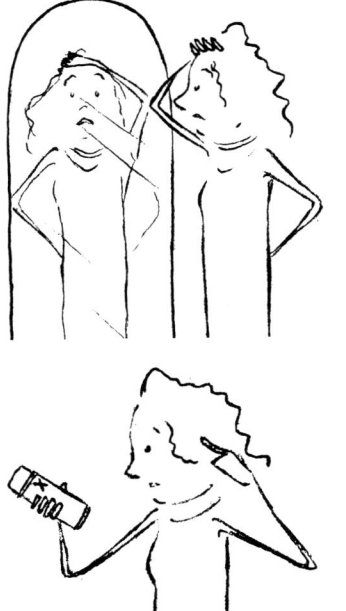

There have been hundreds of versions of this pitch in commercials and ads over the decades, but here is the catch: The product-X manufacturers do not run the following disclaimer, "For Caucasian-type hair only." Why should they? Their miracle product is for everyone with 'normal' hair, isn't it? From the perspective of the majority culture this might be true, but for African Americans, Buffy is clearly not like them. More to the point, African American women are the unspoken, but clearly understood symbolic opposites of

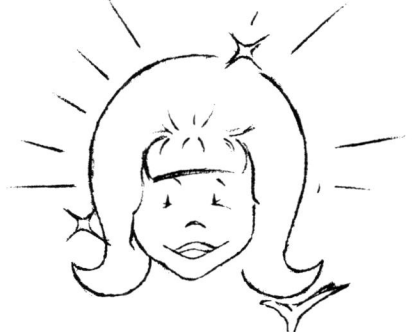

Buffy. They could not have been further from the minds of the product-X manufacturers and promoters when the Buffy image was created. In fact, their (our) inclusion in their thinking would have seemed somehow absurd!

I know this sounds harsh, but it reflects the experiences of millions of African-descended women. Recent efforts of some hair care manufacturers to capture the African American market have not yet successfully reformed this mind set. Our daily lives continue to demonstrate how silence, erasure and denial seem preferable to confronting this harsh reality. Do not think that we haven't tried to BE Buffy. We too would like to forget or ignore the symbolic meanings assigned to our natural hair texture. These meanings affect our self image, and impose limitations to our participation in society.

Yes, these meanings are 'only' symbolic, and there may be no 'real,' concrete limitations at all! Someone may have pleasing features, a deep, lush skin tone, and attractive, beautifully arranged hair. But the negative racial <u>symbolism</u> speaks louder than all of this, making us seem undesirable, or insignificant, or even invisible! By the same token, it is the <u>symbolism</u> of the Buffy image that makes her appearance seem so powerful and valuable.

My mother, like many mothers of her generation, was full of sayings. She would often warn us that actions spoke louder than words. I was very young when I first heard this, and I remember having trouble imagining how actions could 'speak.' Today of course, I do understand what she meant by this, and more. In fact, I could add to my mothers wisdom, by saying that ***Symbols speak louder than words <u>and</u> actions, and for that matter, they often speak louder than concrete physical reality!*** It doesn't matter what we say or do, or what we look like. If the symbolism is not right, then the power of our words and our deeds is weakened.

We know that the symbols operating in our world are often not right for us. This is a most painful reality for African Americans, and it is a source of deep resentment. Considering that we must nonetheless continue to move in this world, we look for ways of making the symbols fit. If the symbols won't change, we will change to fit the symbols. Some would simply call this 'assimilation.' Most anthropologists know that assimilation is an anthropological fact, and has occurred in cultural groups countless times throughout human history. But as long as "blackness" (and all of its negative associations) is defined as the necessary opposite of whiteness (and all of its positive associations) within Western culture, it can **never** be assimilated. Within this framework, there is only room for its subjugation and negation.

So sadly, as long as this racialist framework stands, our transformation (assimilation) can only be a myth of our own creation. Mind you, the product-X people are pleased that we buy into their illusion too, at least for as long as it takes to make a purchasing decision. Judging by the arsenal of hair care products your average African American woman has accumulated in pursuit of that dream, the product manufacturers benefited enormously from our efforts.

In order to be transformed, we must first somehow get our hair into the range of what is considered 'normal.' Since it is our hair <u>texture</u> that puts us beyond the pale of normalcy - at least of the Buffy variety - we try everything we can think of to correct that. Namely, we seek to eliminate all signs of its texture, and behave as though **length**, **style** and **color** were our only concerns. Only then can we play out the rest of the dream, which is simply a version of the American Dream, isn't it? This is one reason we feel entitled to it. This is our dilemma, and we have been grappling with this dilemma for quite a few generations now.

Are we to be faulted for seeking to be normal by the majority culture's standards? Absolutely not! Especially if we consider what the alternative to being normal has meant for African peoples historically. I want to point out here that when I refer to the racialism inherent in Western cultural history, people are often made to feel uncomfortable. "Here comes

> *Are we to be faulted for seeking to be normal by the majority culture's standards? Absolutely not!*

the race card," is the reaction of some, while others feel embarrassment or guilt over the horrors of our past. This is where I find my academic work to be very helpful in convincing people that these are not just the ravings of an angry, uninformed individual with a victim mentality.

For example, I feel it is very important for us to know that for several centuries, racialism (assigning value based on racial characteristics) was an inherent part of the thinking in ALL of the major disciplines of Western Europe. The cultural ancestors of those who colonized the so-called New World took it for granted that physical attributes were outward markers of spiritual quality. Many of the great thinkers who were steeped in these traditions, held what today we would call racist assumptions. These assumptions were so deeply integrated into their thinking that they passed for logical. I go into detail on this in another section, so I'll just cite a brief example here of the kind of thing that is fairly widely known in Africanist, Afrocentric and other academic circles.

In the Western European tradition of philosophy, Immanuel Kant is a tremendously important figure. I would wager that every university philosophy department in this country includes him, or references to his work, on its mandatory reading lists. In one instance, while evaluating the comments of an African-descended individual, Kant remarked that, "... in short, this fellow was quite black from head to foot, a clear proof that what he said was stupid."[2] Imagine the impact of this kind of 'logic' when applied, as it was, on a mass scale.

Now imagine how this kind of thinking must have affected black women of the time? It would certainly have diminished the **truth value** of their roles as legitimate wives and mothers. And of course, to speak of a black woman as beautiful within this way of thinking would have been utterly absurd! Blackness was felt to be the perversion of beauty, truth and virtue.

Overcoming the prevailing negative assumptions about the symbolic meaning of our skin color and hair, has been the greatest obstacle we have had to face as a people worldwide. In this country as most of us know, our history provides us with some of the most graphic examples of the high price we paid for the negative

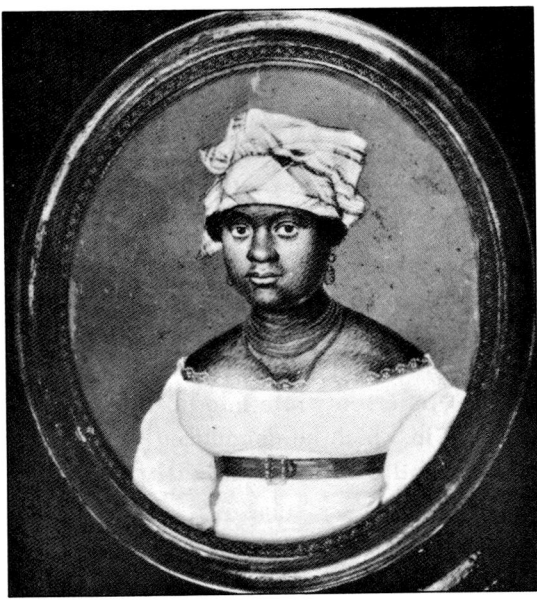
Madame Pierre Toussaint - a respectable black woman of the late 18th century

assumptions of others which often assailed our people. Ironically, most of us today have little understanding of what that challenge meant for our forebearers during the days before Civil Rights, the Black middle class and the straightening comb.

The act of simulating someone else's normality in order to counteract the negativity assigned to the way we looked, was for a long time a survival necessity. This is in part why Buffy continues to hold such a lure for us today. In the past, when a black person's dress, their speech and their hair were <u>not</u> cause for alarm, their chances for access, and ultimately success increased. Though women were generally not perceived as a physical threat to the degree that men were, their hair continued to set them radically apart from the norm. It was therefore seen as an obstacle to be overcome, or at least 'normalized'.

The development of products and techniques that alter the natural characteristics of African-type hair were seen as one way to counteract the devastating impact of society's negative assumptions about blackness. We sought to 'correct' our hair. Corrective technology began developing as early as the last century among African descended slaves who used a combination of lye and vegetable starch to concoct a salve that would straighten their hair. The straightening comb appeared in its crudest form before the turn of the century, and was based on the principle of applying heat and pressure to temporarily remove the tight coils from the hair. This technique became widely popularized, and was in fact much less harmful to the hair than the lye concoction which often caused severe burns and hair loss. There were drawbacks with the straightening comb too, however. It could also burn the hair and scalp, and hair would tend to 'go back' in the presence of water.

Madame C.J. Walker is the name most people associate with what can be thought of as the establishment of the black hair care industry on any scale. She not only perfected the design of the straightening comb, she also developed professional techniques for straightening the hair, and improved formulas for texturizing. Most importantly, she established professional standards for beauticians that are still respected today.

As you can see, there are two sides to our hair care history and the symbols we derive from it. On one side, our efforts represent a courageous fight against tremendous odds to break down barriers to full participation in the mainstream. It has been a fight for the right to assign our own appropriate meanings and values to those important symbols that help us give meaning to our lives. When necessary, we resorted to conformity, because on some level we understood that this was a way of lessening the devastating impact of the extremely powerful symbolic code we were up against.

Although conformity may have increased our chances for survival and success, not surprisingly, there were negative consequences for us as a people when we behaved and made ourselves appear in ways that supported the symbolic systems of others, while weakening our own. The price was paid in our patterns of denial and chronic self-effacement that continue to mark our culture today. Sadly, we have bought into what others had to say about us, and allowed the truth value of our own cultural symbols to be diminished by, or even replaced by other symbols that deny our own unique reality. This paradox stares back at us each time we face our morning grooming and ask, "What will I do with my hair?" When we speak this question, it has an entirely different ring to it than Buffy could ever imagine.

We are living with skeletons in our closets. Though no one alive today is responsible for putting them there, we all inherit the impact of generations of imitation and denial, and of wanting desperately to be 'normal' even when this supposed normalcy is unnatural for us. Somewhere in our heart of hearts, we are aware of this each time we pick up miracle product-X that promises to make our hair 'silky' 'shiny' or 'long'. Our current state of affairs is compounded by a general lack of openness about the kinds of issues I am discussing here. I know of no other group where generations of women do not even know what their natural hair looks like, because from early childhood we routinely alter it or cover it up. I know of no other group whose hair care professionals know so little about their own people's natural hair. The majority of our professionals will not even work with hair that has not been altered by chemicals or heat.

> *I know of no other group whose hair care professionals know so little about their own people's natural hair.*

Because of our past, we have constructed a tradition of hair care based on a fiction; that straight hair is 'normal' for us. As a group, we go to great lengths to simulate someone else's hair-reality. Even the added hair we use to achieve some of our very artful ethnic styles, sends mixed messages because for many, it must be straight hair. We do these things because we want to participate in the majority culture's symbolism of normalcy. In the past this was because of the very painful consequences of not being normal, but today we must take a serious look at this and ask why we continue in this way.

I know that our foremothers did the best they could with what they had. **My own grandmother, in the Walker tradition, proudly referred to herself as a "cosmetologist, specializing in damaged hair" and she was damned good at what she did!** Even into her generation, our women inhabited a world that we today can scarcely understand, and their ability to adapt themselves to its rules was their salvation. When my grandmother was still a girl, Madame C.J. and her contemporaries were somehow making a way out of no way, and because of their successes, my gran had a dignified profession to step into. She went to her grave fiercely proud of the pride and independence this afforded her.

But today, we have reached the stage where we no longer have to adapt

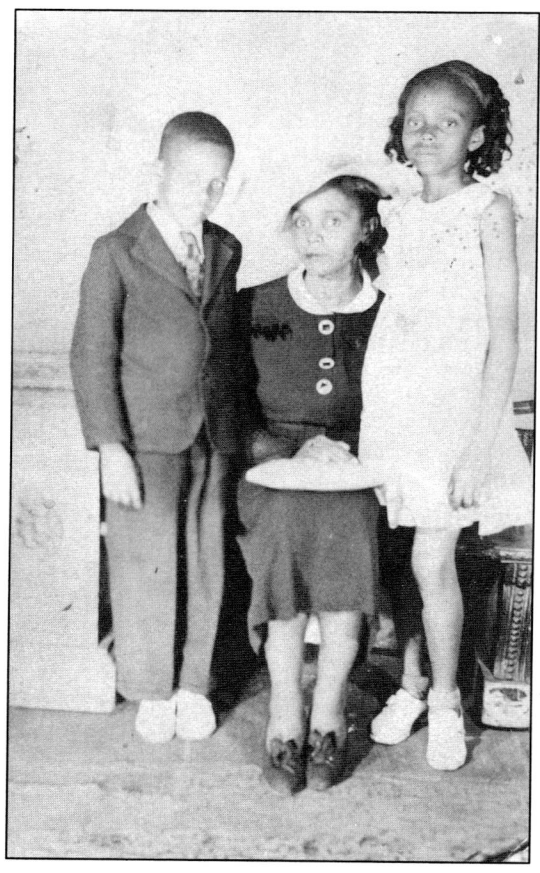

By 1944, grandma was finishing beauty college in Detroit.

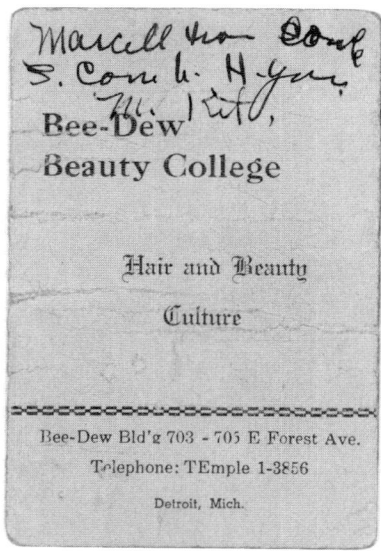

Like many African Americans, Grandma moved her family to Detroit in the 30s for a new life.

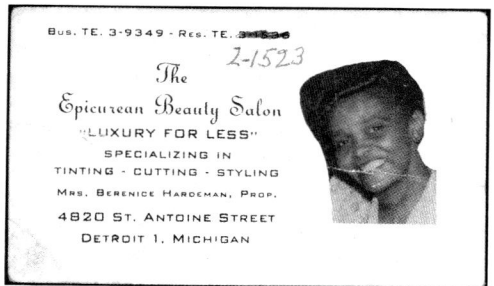

By the early 1950s she owned and operated her own salon.

to the same degree. Those of us who continue, do so out of choice, or habit, or lack of information about other alternatives, or simply fear of exploring un-imagined possibilities.

Our issues are significantly different than those our foremothers faced. Today, no one is making us not accept and celebrate what we really are on any level. We have the ability to set new standards based on our unique and stunning natural attributes, and it is high-time we began seriously asking ourselves what symbols we are wearing on our heads.

1. Standard Textbook of Cosmetology, Israel Rubenstein, ed., (Bronx: Milady Publishing Corporation), 1988, p.221.

2. Race, Writing and Difference, Henry Louis Gates, ed., (Chicago: University of Chicago Press), 1986, p. 11. (Gates is quoting from Immanuel Kant, Observations of the Feeling of the Beautiful and Sublime, translated by John T. Goldthwait (Berkeley and Los Angeles, 1960), p. 111.)

That Hair Thing

Chapter 3
NATURAL HAIR IN THE WORKPLACE

African American women are not newcomers to the workplace in this society. Long before any social movement rallied behind women's right to work outside the home, our women were making daily treks to that side of town where they could be paid for cooking, cleaning and watching over other people's children. We also know that on a fundamental level, there was dignity in this work, DESPITE the fact that not too many decades earlier, this same work had been extracted from our foremothers without pay. Women were serious about the responsibilities their working lives demanded of them. During these times the long-term stability of their situations depended not simply on how well they did their jobs, but also on whether the image projected by their physical appearance was found suitable by their employers. Remember, these women worked primarily for individuals rather than for companies as is the case today. This meant that one person's

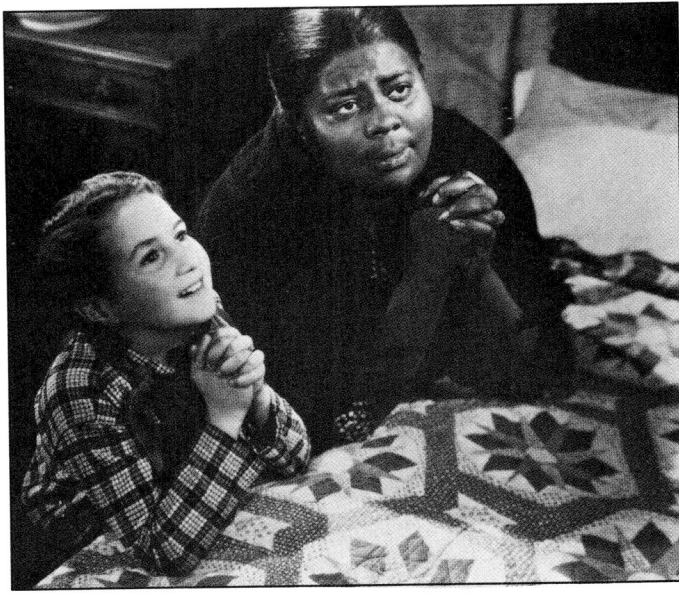

Louise Beavers in one of her many maid roles.

idiosyncrasies, mood swings, changes in personal fortune and so on, impacted directly on their job security from day to day.

Some would even argue that appearances were more important than job skills for domestic workers, and I'm not just talking about neat appearance here either. A specific dress code stood as an assurance that the established order was being upheld. All kinds of popular images reinforced the requirement for subservient appearance during this period when maid (and butler) figures constituted the predominant images of black life in this country. The media stood firmly behind this requirement, and household memorabilia reinforced the same strong message.

I still have vivid memories of my daily walk to elementary school during the '50s that took me through a few blocks of an upper middle class white neighborhood. I felt perpetually embarrassed at all the 'colored' butler and lawn jockey figures and door stops I had to pass along the way. I would occasionally catch a glimpse of one of the real live maids who had somehow allowed herself to get caught by the gaze of us black children. Invariably she wore a formless dress, an apron and shoes which were not designed to accentuate feminine grace. And of course, the hair had to be contained, either in a straight, conservative style with a hair net, or covered completely with a bandanna.

This world that was theirs, but also mine, was full of painful and puzzling contradictions for me. While I knew there was dignity in work and these were 'good' jobs, I always had a feeling of embarrassment upon seeing these maids who also seemed embarrassed to be seen. I attributed this to their needing to hide or camouflage the best parts of themselves for their jobs. I wondered what they were like at home.

Women of my generation have an intimate relationship with those 'maids in America'. These were our mothers and grandmothers. By the time my older sister and I were born, our grandmother had finished her cosmetology training, and was well on her way to owning her own shop. But as a young woman, she was also one of the legions of maids, hard-working and proud. It's hard for me to picture her in any way besides that sassy, independent grandma she was when we knew her. The flair and splash of women like her, their colors and sass,

> *African American women in the work place today are still dealing with the perception that certain things we do make us too ethnic.*

gave life to their homes, but had to be put aside come Monday morning. These women certainly had to keep themselves from being too 'ethnic' in order to get what they needed for their families. We know that the strategies many of them used to 'get over' were not always psychologically healthy, but made it possible for large numbers of young folks - my mother and us included - to live lives free from bitter want, and from the necessity of bowing down before anyone else.

African American women in the work place today are still dealing with the perception that certain things we do make us too ethnic. This, we feel, can threaten our economic stability. These perceptions hit hardest at upwardly mobile, career oriented women, working in private sector jobs where being perceived as threatening is clearly not the way to succeed. You may know of incidents, as I do, where looking too ethnic about the head has actually cost women their jobs. My hat goes off to those women who actually pursued issues like this into the courts, setting precedents for the less courageous among us. Our women have fought against outrageous attitudes and even more outrageous odds to establish our right to define beauty in our own terms. Even more important, their actions challenged people's perceptions of what is 'normal' by insisting that black women not be held to external standards that require us to alter our natural attributes.

Despite individual victories however, the fact remains that most of us are too self conscious, or feel too powerless to go against that unspoken rule that says we must strive to look like what someone else expects us to look like. I don't mean to imply that the majority of our women are simply victims of a system that is generally intolerant of cultural differences. I am in fact amazed at the number of women I have met who have actually taken a stand. But there can be a tremendous amount of stress that goes along with taking a stand. The obstacles are often huge and the payoffs for individual efforts seem so small. In most cases, we feel powerless to change prevailing attitudes no matter what we do, and this results in many of our women feeling deeply frustrated and angry.

Working with my own business over the past several years, I have been immersed in the private sector environment. This has shown me how it is still possible for a single company manager or owner's attitudes and prejudices to shape the policies and practices of small and medium-sized businesses. I have heard women in these environments complain that they still feel like maids in their work place. Typically, the attitudes of these business owners and individuals in management are rife with misconceptions about us as a group. Women working in such environments often deal with significant levels of stress, even (and perhaps especially) when they are trying to conform to what they perceive as acceptable standards of appearance and behavior. In addition to the pressure they may sense from above, they may also feel pressure from co-workers.

Ironically, it may be less stressful when a woman knows which individual or group is responsible for perpetuating negative racial attitudes in the work place. At least in this case she has a target at which to focus her anger. Too often though, this is not the case. When negative attitudes are communicated through very subtle messages coming from a variety of sources, women can actually find themselves internalizing a sense of blame or responsibility for what is perceived as their inappropriateness. They think there is something wrong with them! They become their own harshest critics, at times overly critical of what they believe others find unacceptable about them.

I have seen extreme cases where women act as if they're paranoid about making ethnic statements with their hairdos. They are sure that 'going natural' would be totally unacceptable to their working colleagues, even when they have gotten no clear signals from anyone in particular that this is the case. As I have indicated, there may be

---

I have heard women in these (private sector) environments complain that they still feel like maids in their work place.

grounds for this paranoia. On the other hand, the people around her may actually be indifferent to what she might do to change her appearance. In some cases, they might actually endorse the change. In situations like this however, the women themselves may be creating the uncomfortable feelings through their anxieties about how they think other people might react. They have bought so totally into the idea that their natural appearance is unacceptable, that they can't imagine this not being the case. This is a form of defeatism that kills the urge toward self-exploration and self-empowerment.

Some of you reading this may reply, *"That's fine, but just because I'm paranoid doesn't mean they're not out to get me!"* This is true, but at the core - and this is key - I don't believe that the aversion to natural hair we experience on a mass scale as African American women, is really due primarily to our concern about upward mobility, our bosses' attitudes or our jobs. If this were the case, we would expect to find an abundance of natural hair styling among women whose jobs are not at stake.

The fact is that even when our women experience little or no pressure to conform to specific hair styling codes because of issues in the work place, we find straight styles predominating, and sharp negative attitudes about our own natural hair types. Even when women have lifestyles where they are expected to be ethnic, often their beautifully braided styles continue to communicate a subtle message of dependence on the straight hair look. My casual survey of women from all of these groups shows that they are equally as likely to scorn their natural hair. In some cases there may be little or no pressure coming from the work place, but there is pressure nonetheless in their lives that informs their choices. The message comes through loud and clear from their families, from their churches, from their significant-others and peers. Nobody wants to see, much less wear their natural hair.

I have carried out my casual survey far and wide, and from what I have been able to determine, this attitude cuts across all age, class and geographical barriers. The message that our natural, African-type hair is simply wrong has been uttered for so long and so effectively that women - and men - from all walks of life have bought into the myth.

> *The message that our ... hair is simply <u>wrong</u> has been uttered for so long and so effectively that women - and men - from all walks of life have bought into the myth.*

I have had women tell me about how they were turned away at the doors of their church by their pastors when they tried to wear their hair naturally. I have had women describe to me the reactions of their own young children who, seeing them for the first time in their natural hair, reacted in fright. I have heard from women who as young girls were made to wear wigs because a parent couldn't relate to or manage their natural hair.

The bottom line is that though <u>some</u> of us must cope with work place related pressures, for the most part, the significant pressures we experience come from much closer to home. Let's face it, they DO come from home!

From my perspective, these home-based negative attitudes are by far the most insidious and detrimental. While there are laws today against practicing discrimination on the job, there are not yet any laws against practicing self-denigration and perpetuating self-hatred at home. Nonetheless, we must start acting as though such laws exist, because these attitudes are like crimes we commit against ourselves and those we claim to love. Our own negative attitudes surface in many ways, but one area I find most challenging is how they create discontinuity in our lives. We lose perspective on the dangers these negative attitudes foster when their source is so close to the heart. As a result, we develop the ability to live lives full of glaring contradictions.

Imagine what would happen if your daughter's white third grade teacher routinely and openly made culturally insensitive comments in class about her ethnic-looking hair. You would probably, rightfully, try to have that teacher's job! Most of us are pretty good at recognizing this brand of racism. But would we display the same righteous indignation if the offender were the deacon of our church? ("Sister, you know I love you and your family like my own, but sister, that's no way for a child to be lookin'!"); Or when the offender is our mother who is constantly offering to pay for that kiddy-perm; Or when the offender is our boy child who, as he develops more and more street-savvy, is already helping her feel that her hair will be wrong no matter what she does to it?

Make no mistake about it, these are crimes against the person just as surely as if that person were being victimized by racist attitudes on the job, though all the more painful because they come from loved ones. These negative attitudes are one of the most tragic outcomes of our historical victimization. Tragically, they bear testimony to racism's triumph over our lives by making racists of its victims. Once this has been accomplished, there is no longer any need for outside agitation, we continue to do ourselves in!

The problem is huge in our communities, we know this. How will we resolve it? It seems to me that this will occur not by focusing on the symptom or result of the problem - that is, our preference for straight hair. Instead, we must find ways to focus on its causes. For example, many of us still perceive the need for continued self-effacement as a way to survive and thrive within the majority culture. This don't-stand-out syndrome can be taken to an unhealthy extreme though. When this is the case, internalized racism is surely at work. How do we know when we've reached this unhealthy level? To be sure, that is an individual call, but if you're like the many African American women I know who are ready to take an uzi into work to equalize their frustration over having to conform, I'd say it's time to get more self-critical, and ask what is going on at the deeper levels!

Being self-critical is an approach to resolving our problems that carries my full endorsement. Let's look at ourselves honestly and ask what is keeping us from confronting the unhealthy influences in our lives. Along with that I recommend cultivating self-love, learning self-acceptance and unlearning the 'victim mentality' that immediately causes us to assume that "they" are after us. This seems to be one of the most pernicious forms of social malaise our people suffer. Follow the examples of women (and men) like you, who are acting on their intention to find their way back to a solid cultural foundation. I have discovered that despite what we are told, there is no shortage of role models by which to set our course.

For me, the task of unlearning the victim mentality has been an act of love and a journey back to myself. As I began to reconnect, I found I was no longer capable of looking at myself through the eyes of a disapproving 'other'. Not only that, I discovered that **I** became the one who was setting the standards for those around me to follow. This was true in my work environment as well as at home and in my local community. The same has happened to many women who have made the journey back to themselves. And by the way, they still have their jobs.

Most of us who were not born perfect, don't remember when or how we became lost to ourselves, or at what moment the lush beauty of our skin, our form and our hair began to fade from our perception. That's because this didn't happen in our lifetime. It is part of the legacy we inherited from our difficult cultural past. Though we're not responsible for creating the problem we are responsible for ending it by re-clarifying our perception of ourselves. I often think of that line in Maya Angelou's poem, "And Still I Rise". It reads:

"I am the dream and the hope of the slave"

That line really does something to me. I imagine my foreparents literally trying to make a way out of no way, having to make undreamed of compromises that took a devastating toll on their self esteem and psychological well being. I imagine that what is keeping them going is the dream that one day, long after they imagine themselves dead and gone, I will be born - **Me!** And I will be the one to finally set things right in their name. They're counting on me, and that thought gives them strength. I guess you might say that I draw my strength from my vision of my foreparents' belief in me. They made it over because in their dreams, I made it over too!

I take this as my legacy, and it seems to balance all of the negative energy from their past and my own. I am, **we are** their victory! When we look at our lives in this way, we've already won. We don't have to wear 'the uniform' anymore - not at home and not in the work place. We can love ourselves openly and wear our unique natural beauty proudly. **We have made it over.**

Some Who Have Made It Over:

Genitha

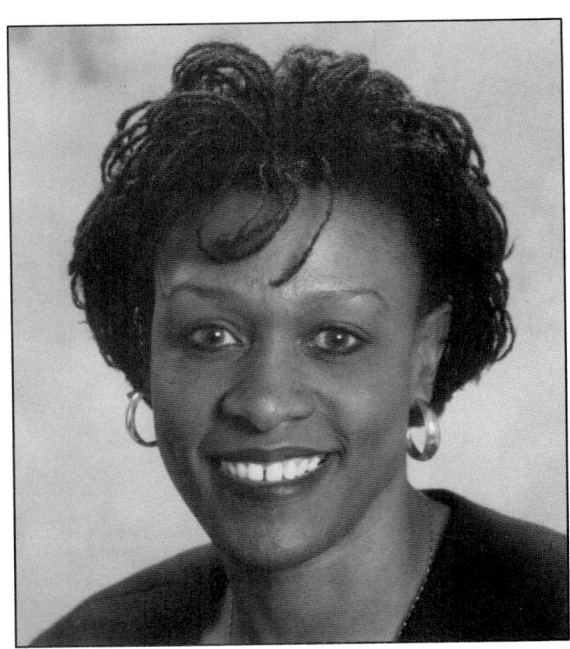

Occupation:
Secretary - Public Works Office

Time in Locks:
1 year

Reactions in the Work Place:
"People don't understand natural hair. After a year, I still get the same questions." "I get positive comments, and some friendly joking comments too, mostly by non-blacks. Black women just look, wanting to say something, but they don't." "Getting locks was not a big deal for me. The confidence I show in wearing them doesn't allow people to put me down."

54 That Hair Thing

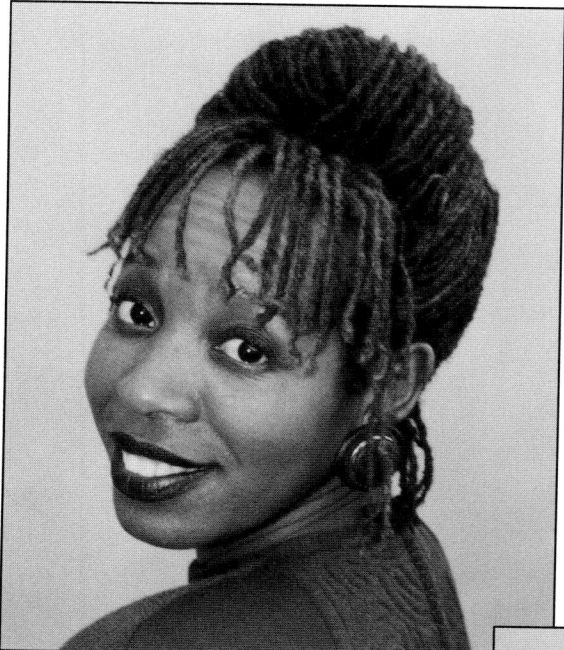

Eleane

Occupation:
Licensed Insurance Agent and Trainer

Time in Locks:
15 Months

Reactions in the Work Place:
"Very positive from regional president on down." "They can't imagine me without locks. I think It has caused them to respect me even more as a black woman ... because I'm proud of my heritage."

Anne

Occupation
Offset Press Operator

Time in Locks
1 Year, 9 Months

Reactions in the Work Place:
"I had worn an Afro for about 15 years prior to getting the locks." "Many people assumed they were dreads. They asked me a lot of questions" "I was a little uncomfortable at first, but that wore off."

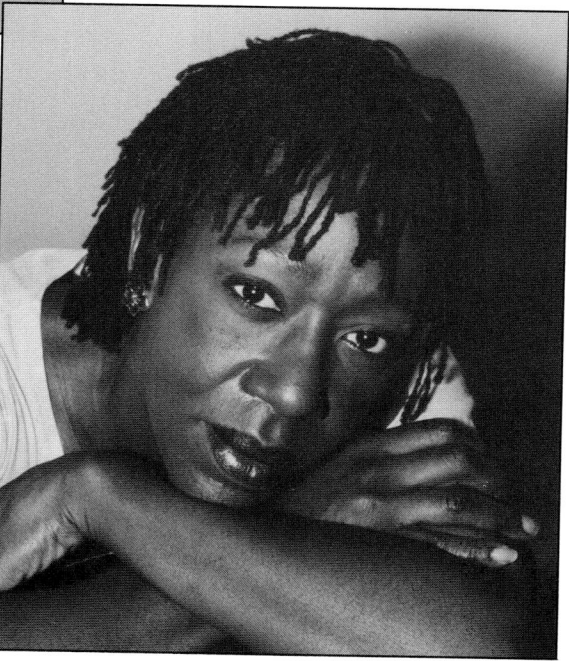

Elorse

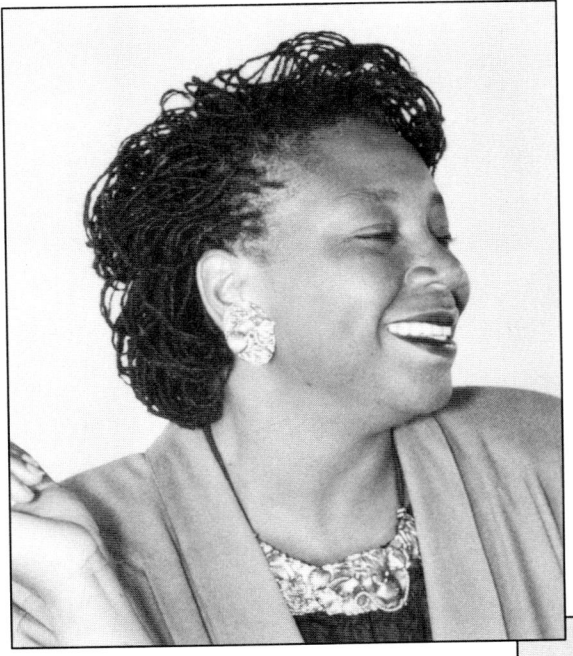

Occupation:
Probation Officer

Time in Locks:
2 years

Reactions in the Work Place:
"I had worn braids a long time. Once I got locks I was so proud to have my own hair, I didn't care what others thought." "It's not really about making a statement. It's just us accepting ourselves as opposed to them accepting us!" "This is me! I have more self-pride"

Linda G.

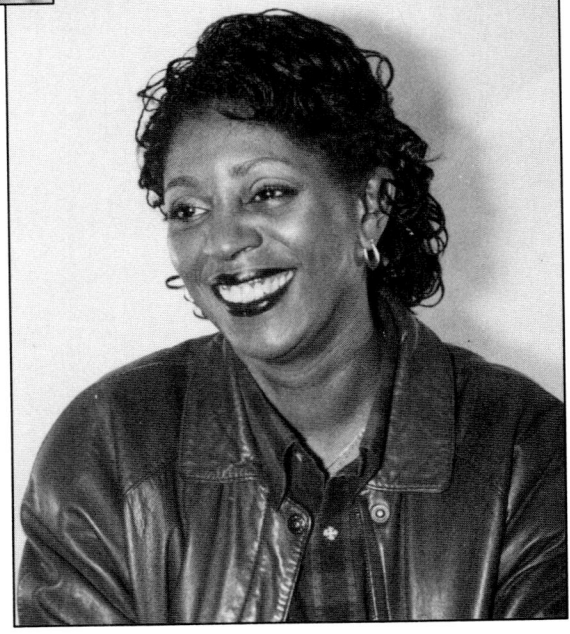

Occupation:
Electronic/Mechanical Assembly Worker

Time in Locks:
6 Months (Transitioning from relaxer)

Reactions in the Work Place:
"The reactions were positive, but I wasn't really concerned about reactions. To each his own." "A person ought to do what they want to do" "I like natural hair. It's much easier."

56 That Hair Thing

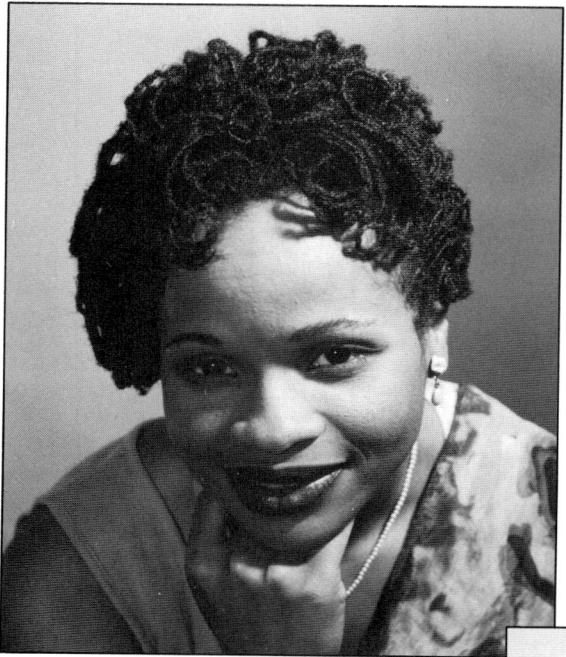

Linda R.

Occupation:
Bankruptcy Clerk for Chapter 13 Trustee

Time in Locks:
1 Year

Reactions in the Work Place:
"I work with about 20 people. I get compliments from all different kinds of people." "Some people think my locks will create a promotional problem in corporate America. I guess if that's the way they judge me, the job isn't worth it!"

Alice

Occupation:
Singer

Time in Locks:
2 1/2 Years

Reactions in the Work Place:
"The overall response has been remarkable." "I'm always meeting people who want to know what the locks are and how they can get them."

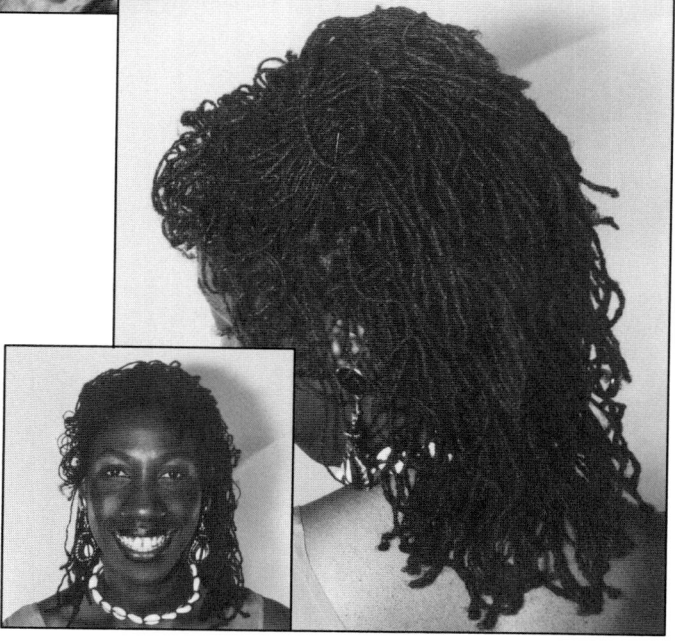

Natural Hair In The Workplace   57

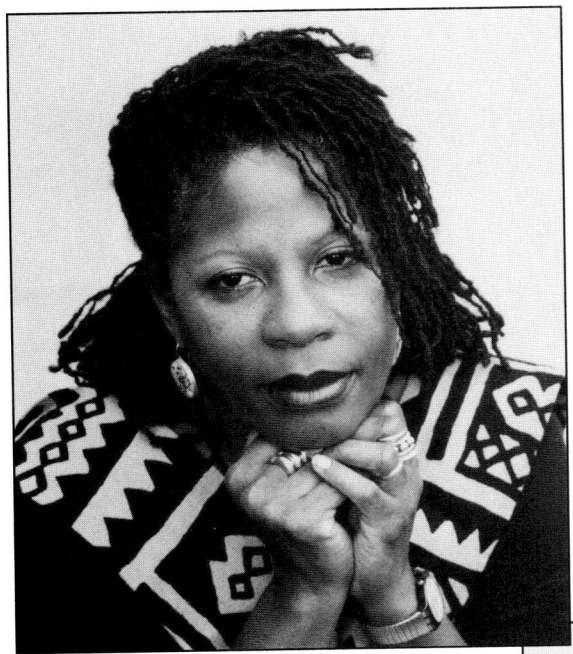

Annis

Occupation:
Director of Providor Network Services (HMO)

Time in Locks:
3 Years

Reactions in the Work Place:
"I wondered if my locks would be accepted. At first it drew a few double takes." "Questions were asked, and I got more attention. They haven't been an obstacle though" "I wouldn't go back to relaxers to get a new job." "People say it's not for them. I say once you accept yourself it works for you too."

Wanda

Occupation:
Student Services Case Manager (Public Schools)

Time in Locks:
2.5 Years

Reactions in the Work Place:
"I tried to prepare people for what I was going to do, but they all thought I would look like Whoopi!" "I got mixed reactions. The young **men** liked it but not all of the women did. As my locks grew and filled in, comments all turned positive." "Being confident in myself as a black person helped me through the transition."

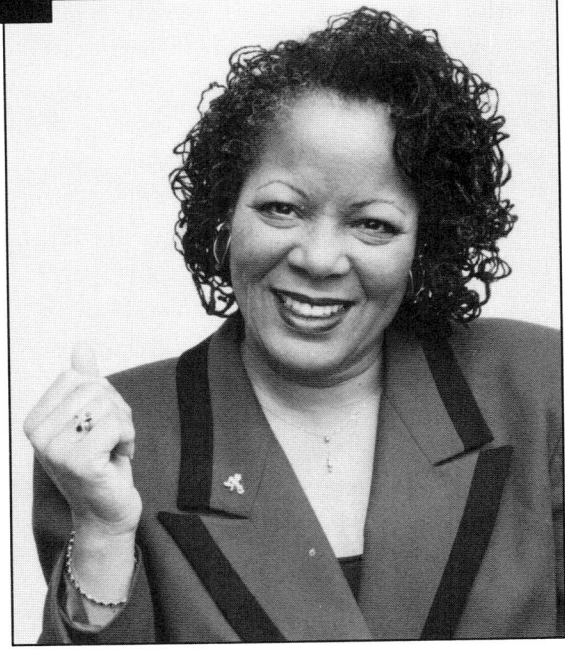

58 That Hair Thing

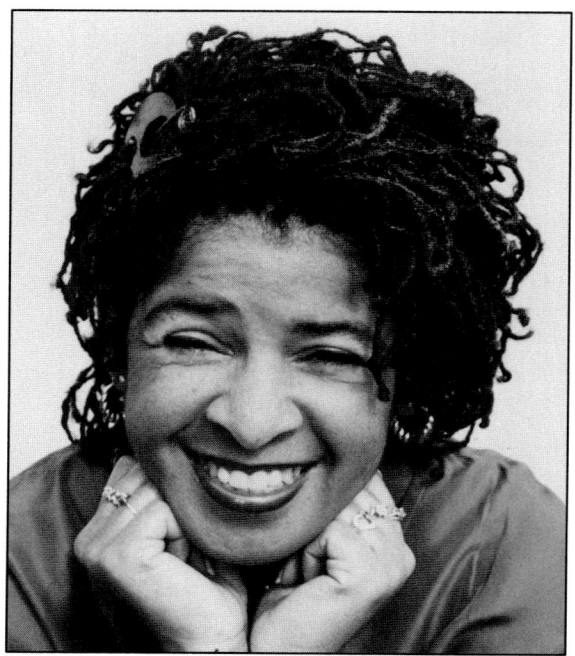

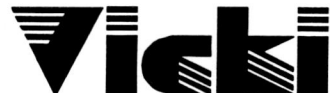

Occupation:
Engineering Cost Associate

Time in Locks:
3 Years

Reactions in the Work Place:
"When I told my co-workers I was getting locks they were not enthusiastic. They asked why, and said I looked fine the way I was." "When I got them everyone was really curious and wanted to touch it. Most like it." "They are amazed by the versatility. Every time I wear a new style they think it's been re-done!" "Even co-workers who were skeptical at first are coming around."

Snarls

**by
Jane Milligan**

I keeps my hair short, natural.

Don't feel like jerkin' comb through
    snarls of history,
        knots of pain.

I keeps it manicured
    like a neat lil' bush--
        weekly trims 'round edges,
            daily dabs of oil
                to soothe the roots.

Other day
    gave myself a summer trim.
        Hair felt cool,
            looked neat,
                combed quick.

Next day
    coworker, white, seemed painfully
        perplexed
            'bout the status of my hair;
                was vital for her to know,
                    so she asked.

"Oh," I answered,
    "cut it, myself."
        and furthermore, I implied,
        I preferred it that way.

Thought I put her mind to rest,
    but somthin' still hung
        in the air.

Her eyes bounced everywhichway--
    my head
        my chin
            the walls
                my head again.

The awkward pause
    she finally shoved aside
        with limp remark, "looks nice"...

UMMMMMM HMMMMMMM ...
Failed that lie detector test!
I know.
        I seen the same Clairol commercials
            she has...
                an' then some.

(copyright 1997: Jane Milligan)

That Hair Thing

Chapter 4
A CONSPIRACY OF SILENCE

Is that really your hair? Does it hurt to do that? Can you wash it? It must take forever to do that to your hair! Why do you always change your hair? How do you get that out? Does your hair really grow that fast?

How many of us who have ever worn extensions or twists or locks have NOT heard these questions? Very few, I'll bet! Our hair type and the wide variety of artful ways we wear it, are truly a puzzlement to the majority of Americans. At the same time, these types of questions are a source of irritation for many of our women who typically do not like to be put on the spot about their appearance, and especially about their hair!

There is a lack of meaningful communication about cultural and physical differences in our society. This is partly to blame for why our women so often find themselves put on the spot about the ways they choose to wear their hair. I think it goes further than this though. There has been a conspiracy of silence surrounding our hair type for a very long time; several centuries, in fact. Though this conspiracy has been mainly perpetuated by others throughout history, today African American women also uphold it. Why is that? Here is one perspective:

One of the assumptions of emancipation was that African Americans would finally be blessed with upward mobility within the American social order. Literacy rates soared as our people flocked to school rooms to get

> *There has been a conspiracy of silence surrounding our hair type for a very long time; several centuries, in fact.*

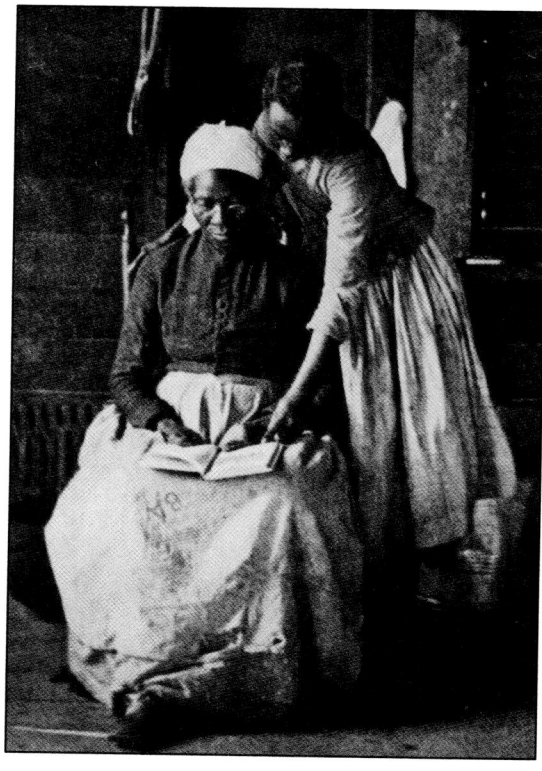

their "learnin'." With inclusion in the American dream as their goal, it soon became clear to former slaves that upward mobility often depended on their willingness to minimize those parts of themselves deemed unacceptable by the majority culture. Unlike today when affirming differences is becoming an acceptable practice, during post-emancipation America, "self-erasure" for many African descended people was to become an important key to survival.

Many of us today still hold on to values that say, "Don't call attention to your differences," though our survival no longer depends on this posture. While everyone knows that our hair is not the same as other types, it is still generally unacceptable in our culture to dwell on, or openly display what makes our hair different. We let others think that there are no issues here, when in truth, within our own communities, hair is a tremendously charged topic.

Because our values shy away from physical expressions of our cultural uniqueness, this has gotten in the way of our own understanding of that uniqueness. We don't want to draw attention to something that we haven't really fully come to terms with yet ourselves. So, this chapter asks some of the thorny, uncomfortable questions, like; "What are the meanings assigned to naturally-textured hair?" "Where did these come from?" "What is it about these meanings that continues to make hair such a closed topic for African American women?"

Let's start by looking closer at the conspiracy of silence I referred to earlier. I use this term because I feel that most of us knowingly avoid talking openly and truthfully about our hair issues. This is usually because it makes us feel vulnerable by exposing our inadequacies. Though our hair issues are of such a magnitude that they affect every aspect of our lives, we allow them to go unresolved, or simply deny they exist. This conspiracy tends to be particularly active in settings where African Americans aren't very numerous; corporate board rooms; dorms at predominantly white colleges; among mainstream public or media figures, and the like. But it might surprise you to learn that the conspiracy is extremely powerful in the arena where our own hair care professionals work and are trained.

In traveling to some of these places to demonstrate my system of natural hair care I have been struck by what can only be described as a bizarre fiction that seems to dominate people's thinking. It is a fiction based on a near-total denial of the obvious: **Our hair type is <u>naturally</u> highly-textured, <u>not</u> straight.** But what is <u>natural</u> is not necessarily considered <u>normal</u> in these environments. In fact, from what I can tell, our natural hair is hardly even discussed among traditionally trained professionals.

What are the reasons behind all this secrecy about our hair? What is it that the world is not supposed to know about us?

You would think that if someone wanted to know the real deal about natural black hair types and care, the best place to look for answers would be in the professional hair care arena. Would it surprise you to learn that most students in beauty schools and cosmetology departments **never** have the opportunity to take even one course dealing with natural, African-type hair care and maintenance? Mind you, these are the people who are preparing to become licensed cosmetologists, and are required to take close to 2,000 hours of professional training. This scenario is the same regardless of whether the students or instructors are African Americans. The silent treatment surrounding our natural hair type has been so fully institutionalized that a beauty college or traditional black beauty salon is probably the **LAST** place you would go to pierce through the veil of secrecy.

When I walk into these environments with my locks, I walk in from another world, one that many are not yet prepared to accept. I usually get the feeling that, just by wearing locks, I am letting a 'dreaded' skeleton out of a closet that many feel a desperate need to keep bolted shut. There is a feeling of uneasiness because no one knows what this skeleton will do once it gets out! The uneasiness I am referring to of course comes from the horrors of our cultural past. There are good reasons why 'That Hair Thing' for African Americans (like skin color) brings up deep self-identity issues. There are also profound reasons why others throughout history have been discouraged from understanding or valuing our differences.

One thing I consistently notice in my interactions with our women is the negative ways we refer to our natural hair. As a reflection of our self-image, this is really disturbing. *Terms such as "kinky," "nappy," "fuzzy," "excessively curly," or get this one, "cainchy-comb-me" (from "can't you comb me?") are used almost exclusively. There is such a lack of positive reference to our natural hair type that it is truly shocking.* We should know that throughout history, our hair has been likened by others to animal wool, burrs, and the like. In fact, nowhere in the literature of Western civilization do you find positive references to African-textured hair.

While I can understand the desire on the part of many African American women to change their hair type to avoid this very old stigma, these negative comments have the opposite effect on some. A growing number of women (and men) are all the more determined not to buy into the straight hair myth. Once someone comes to understand our natural hair type in all its glory, they see that "kinky" doesn't begin to describe the lushness and versatility of it.

It is unfortunate that most of us are unaware of our own rich inheritance of hair artistry that comes to us from the West African cultures. My sense is that this would certainly

> *One thing I consistently notice in my interactions with our women is the negative ways we refer to our natural hair.*

serve to counteract the negativity felt in our daily lives. I have looked into some of the meanings assigned to African-type hair in different times and cultural settings, and found that under normal circumstances, adornment systems, including those for hair, <u>always</u> have very systematic, positive meanings. But what happens when a group's ability to assign appropriate positive meaning is eroded, or co-opted, or simply taken away? What are we left with as a people, with no frame of reference or guide to finding one?

I refer to hair as an adornment, but don't think that it carries only superficial meanings. The way we wear our hair makes statements about who we think we are, and how we see ourselves fitting into our society. It also is a way of responding to conditions around us. Those conditions may promote self expression, or they may encourage conformity, or they may be oppressive. Here I agree with Alice Walker, it is possible to have "oppressed hair."

What do you suppose things were like before black women's hair got oppressed? This state is hard for many of us to imagine, I know, because there is so little in our shared experience that places value on our natural hair types. As a way to gain insight into this, I began looking for information about how women wear their hair in some of the West African regions. Non-European hair styling traditions can still be found in rural areas and smaller communities where people still value and maintain links with their particular cultural histories. What I learned was quite astonishing. The precision with which these women use hair styling to construct meaningful statements about themselves and their place in the world is dazzling! At times playful, or political, or ceremonial, their styles are articulate expressions of their cultural personality.

In Mali for example, there are several ethnic groups where women's hair styling traditions continue to be used very artfully, and carry important positive meanings. Bambara, Khasso, Tamasheq, Peulh, Moorish and Toucouleur women of that nation skillfully express their beauty through the symbolism of their natural hair.

Here is an example of some of the traditions that are still lively today: Young girls must gain a certain age before earning the right to grow their hair for braiding. Once this honor is

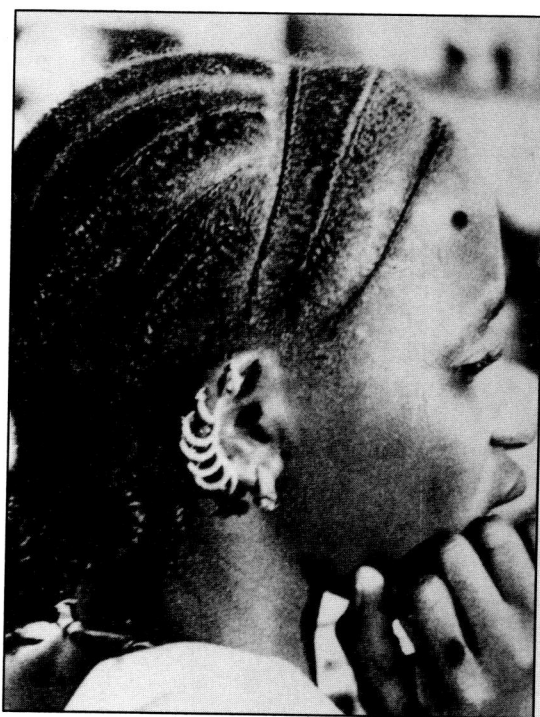

Bambara coiffure for young girls

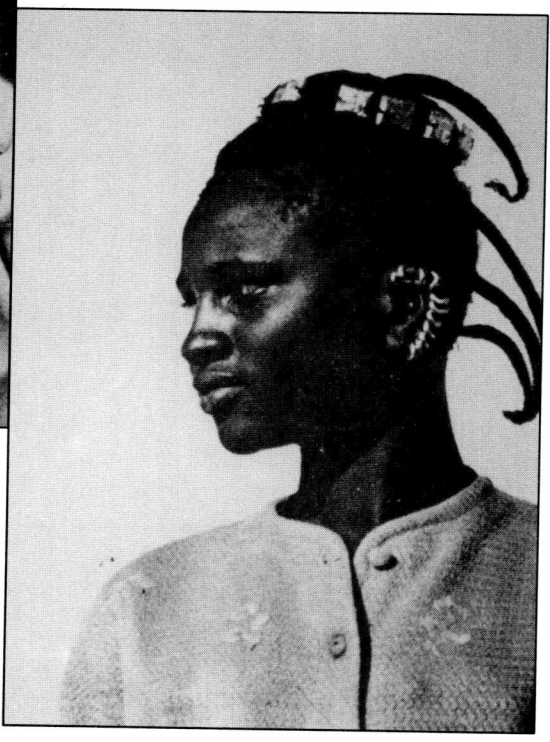

Khasso style for young women - Sends a message that repels negative energy from the wearer's space.

bestowed at about age 7, they gain access to a wide, but very specific range of styles that are determined appropriate to their age group. Once eligible for courting, a new range of options opens up. The intricate hairstyles of this phase can be adorned with a variety of objects whose messages range from coquettishness to spiritual protection to ostentatious displays of wealth.

As a woman matures, the range of hair styling messages deepens to

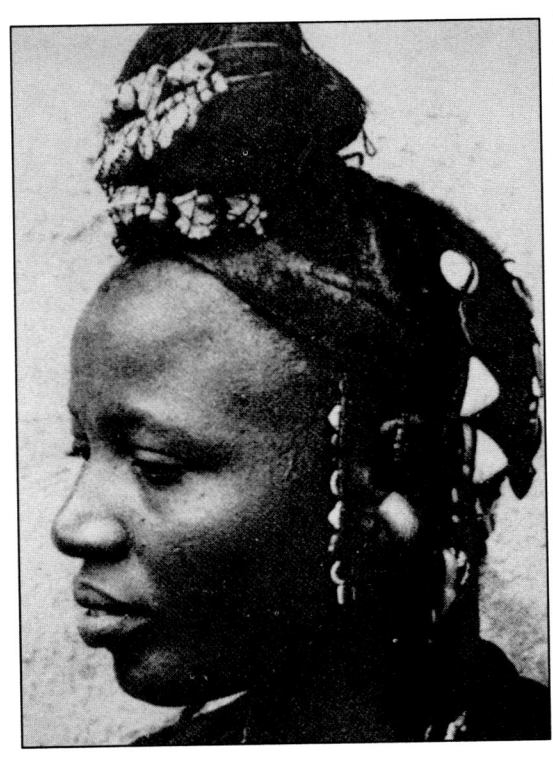

Mature Moorish "beauty" hair style

include expressions of spirituality, political orientation, as well as marital and class standing.

This way of incorporating hair styling choices into the integrated fabric of culture has been the norm for as far back as anyone can remember.

How did the ways of making statements with our hair in our original cultures - positive statements about ourselves and our world - get reduced to one really crass, brutalizing message? This message was imprinted in our cultural psyche long ago, and still remains in some form today: "Our hair type is a visible indication that we are inferior beings." Though it took several generations to take hold, the negative transformation caused by this message has so thoroughly cast its shadow over us, that most today do not even believe there could ever have been a good side to our 'bad' hair. Here is a bit of history that will help put that negative transformation into context:

The systems, or patterns of knowledge that developed in Western Europe as it was becoming dominant in the world, tended to categorize groups of people according to their physical attributes. The so-called sciences of physiognomy and phrenology provide excellent examples of this. In these views, physical traits were taken as indicators of mental and moral capacity, and these in turn were equated with spiritual value, or lack of value, as the case may be.

Quite literally, a person's

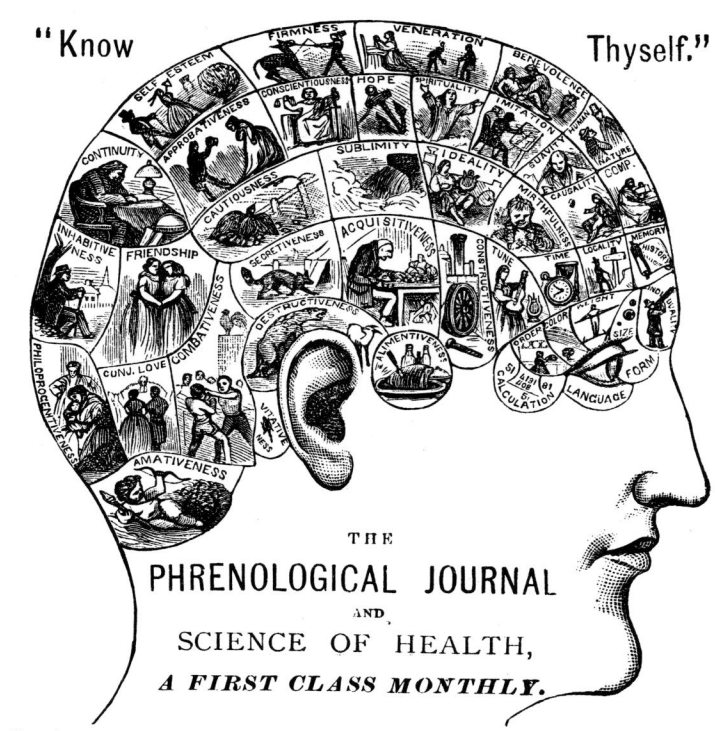

physique, facial features, hair and skin were believed to reflect qualities like virtue, honesty and courage, as well as their opposites. The value assigned to physical traits determined the place of an individual or group within a hierarchy of cultural groups ascending from the animal world below, to the realm of the angels above. The quality of a person's soul was felt to be reflected to some extent in their features. Mind you, this system was not invented just for the exclusion of people of color. It developed primarily out of the ways European cultures viewed each other.

This vision of life on earth was

A typical phrenology head from an 1866 primer on how to 'read' moral, spiritual and intellectual qualities based on physical features.

A Conspiracy of Silence

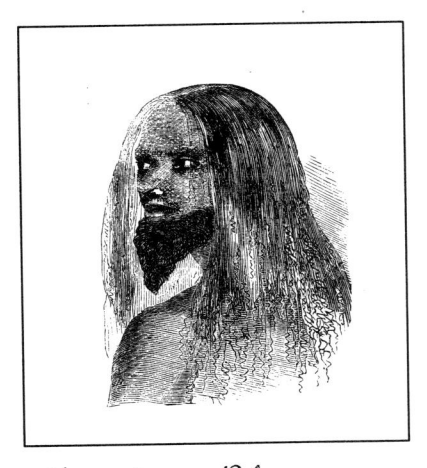

Harawauky man - Polynesia

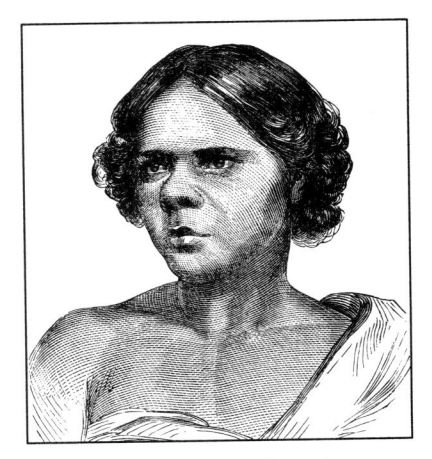

Man of North Australia

derived from, and strengthened by various interpretations of the bible, which at one time was felt to contain all possible knowledge about life on earth.

The problem was that once European explorers began pressing beyond known geographical boundaries, they began encountering groups of people that the bible did not seem to account for. This was troubling since the bible was taken by most to be

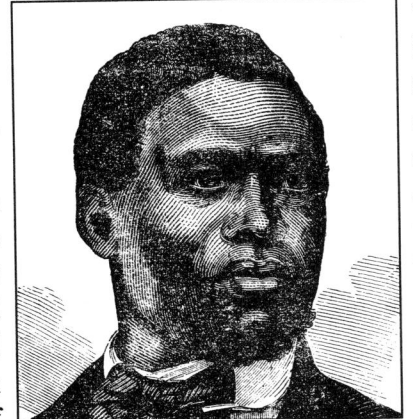

A Negro

the <u>complete</u> story of creation. Encounters with groups whose language, dress, habits and physical appearance were very different, set off several centuries of intense debate about what it meant to be human. Those who assumed that the bible had to be literally true had difficulty accepting that the original couple - Adam and Eve - could have been the ancestors of people who were so different, especially in the case of black skinned people who, according to this logic, had to be at the opposite end of the human spectrum from whites.

In an effort to arrive at an explanation that still allowed for a literalistic interpretation of the bible, several quite elaborate theories emerged to account for these differences. These theories ranged from ones proposing more than one Genesis, to those that suggested a curse was responsible for the supposed ungodly-looking dark skin, snout-like noses and woolly hair of African descended peoples. These attributes were thought to place them near the extreme end of the chain of being, the end closest to the animal world.

Perhaps the most widely accepted of these curse theories was the Curse of Ham. As we know, this curse theory was not simply used to explain difference, but also to justify enslaving Africans and transporting them to an alien world where it was believed by many that they would benefit from their exposure to the 'light' of Christian civilization. Some went so far as to suggest that in this environment, if they were accepting of God's grace, these dark peoples might even turn white!

The views I am describing were by no means random ones expressed by a few crazy individuals. They were consistently expressed by dominant voices for generations in the debate that was carried on within European religious, political and intellectual circles over the nature and proper place of each of the world's peoples. This debate was not just about the suspected inferiority of Africans. It went further, using physical attributes as would-be proof in the debate over whether African and other non-European people were even the same <u>species</u> as European-type people.

This debate carried into our own national history, particularly in discussions surrounding the abolition of slavery. Here is a quote from the arguments of an anti-abolitionist writer of the last century. Consider that this would have been a viable argument at the time: ***"The black colour of negroes, thick lips, flat nose, crisped woolly hair, and rank smell***

> *The views I am describing were by no means random ones expressed by a few crazy individuals.*

distinguish them from every other race of men, ... we argue that these distinct peculiarities of the negroe are characteristics of another species, differing vastly and very essentially from white men."[1] These views (from the curse theory to the polygenesis theory) have been incredibly enduring, and continue to show up into this century. One has only to recall the benchmark legal cases fought and won by the NAACP during the 50s and 60s (i.e. Brown vs. Board of Education) and later, the challenges made by citizens groups against discriminatory licensing requirements in government agencies, the trades and in unions, that were being used to prolong segregation.

Some of the other theories as to why African-type peoples have certain unique attributes seem even more far-fetched than those deriving from the biblical curse idea. Here are a few of the more creative ones:

The mother of the first black person was white, but was frightened while pregnant, and the child was born black; There was widespread disease, and those who survived were left with black skins; Black people

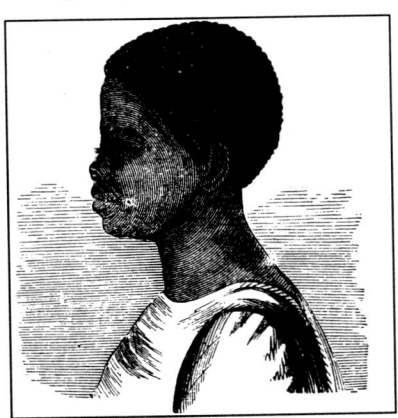

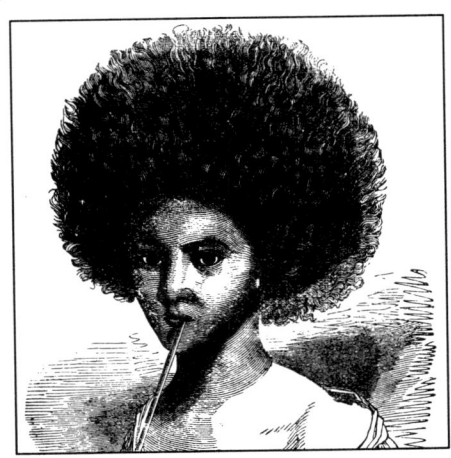

The nose of this "Ethiopian" (black) woman was believed to show development in the direction of deformity, that is, towards the snouts of lower animals.

The hair of this mixed racial woman (Indian and Negro) furnished an example of the "practical jokes which nature sometimes perpetuates in her more playful moods."[2]

descended from a race of animals that resembled humans; Ordinary people (or in some versions, careless savages) were burned by the climate in which they lived, which made them black, and singed their hair, making it appear more like wool.

I know it is painful to dredge up negative cultural references in this kind of detail. However, I need to make it very clear that this kind of thinking laid the foundation for our society today. Though many African Americans (and others) may have suspected that the racialist foundations of our culture ran very deep, it is rare that the kind of information I am touching on here is ever taught in schools, or covered in documentaries or widely circulated in any form. Though we don't openly talk about the negative racial attitudes on which our culture was based, they have been deeply encoded in our culture on every level.

I find that even some of my university colleagues are unaware of the pervasiveness of these past attitudes and teachings, and certainly of the negative impact these have had on African decended people. This is true despite the fact that it is not difficult to document the things I am sharing with you. The people who thought this way and acted on their beliefs were not usually considered monsters in their time, as might be the case today. In fact, they might easily have been in the majority within their groups at the time they wrote.

I want to make two points about all of these theories that sought to explain what our physical differences meant. Notice first the assumption that African humanity is the obvious expression of something that has gone <u>wrong</u> with nature. It is as though we represented the threat of cosmic disorder, and that our physical traits were a constant reminder of that threat. Second is the silence, or erasure of African people within the international debate about them: The objects of this debate had no voice whatsoever in the matter. This last fact alone speaks volumes to me about the profound silencing effect these

---

I need to make it very clear that this kind of thinking laid the foundation for our society today.

attitudes had for the victims. We are still struggling to find our voice today.

Fortunately, as a result of about 150 years of social pressure and about 40 years of legislation, the legacy of this centuries-old view of African humanity is diminishing. However, it remains very much a part of our cultural inheritance. Though the meaning of having naturally-textured hair <u>today</u> may have an ambiguous feel to it, there was very little ambiguity in the past, and our foreparents had to cope with that clear meaning. The message said to them that they were of a race beyond the pale of salvation, and their lives were legislated for them around that 'fact.' They felt the impact of their physical appearance every day, in where they could go, what they could do in life, with whom they could interact, their legal rights (if they had any), and the condition of their souls. Their intellectual capacities, their ability to tolerate pain or experience emotions, were also evaluated based on the same set of assumptions about what their appearance meant.

What has been the effect of all of this on African descended women ? on our ideas about our physical appearance? on our willingness, or even our ability to express those feelings? What is it like to be born into a world where you CANNOT be beautiful (or even acceptable) in your natural state because your soul is cursed, and your skin and your hair are the marks of your degradation? In past generations a woman may even have been told that this was the will of God, and she should simply accept it. In practical terms, there was very little an individual woman could do at that time, except cope as best she could, and accept the obvious fact that beauty was not her birthright.

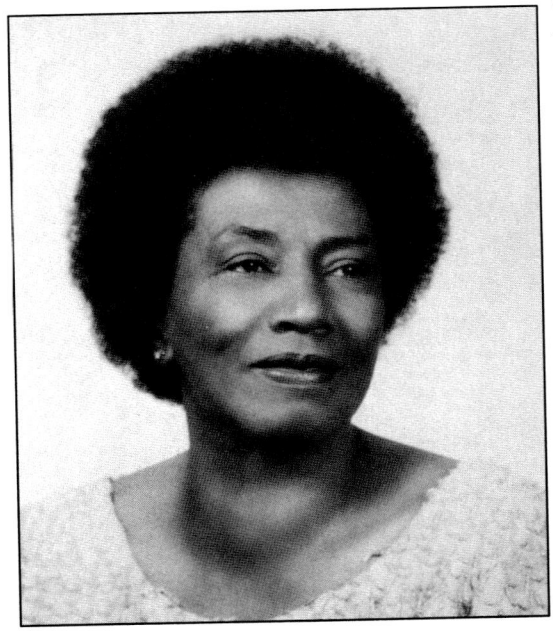

Despite the obstacles, women like composer, pianist amd educator Undine Smith Moore wore their unaltered beauty like a crown.

Though times have changed, African American women still feel the pain of past wounds. This is what so many of us feel, but have no words to express. We had no say in assigning the meanings our hair continues to have within this culture. Nobody asked us what we considered beautiful, or meaningful, or acceptable. We were just told. The tragic irony is that we have lived in that silence for so long, many of us have forgotten how to claim beauty and meaning for ourselves. The weight of that oppressive history, felt in a million subtle ways, took away our voice, and in our frustration, we are likely to snap unnecessarily at the first unsuspecting white person who asks a naive question about our hair.

It's time to start talking, ladies! Talk to 'them', to each other, to our boards of cosmetology, to our media, to our pastors and educators, to our children, to our parents, to our men. Most importantly, it's time to acknowledge that ALL of the feelings we have about our hair are absolutely valid. We didn't create this monster, we are only its victims. But because of our silence, it has grown to be much bigger than life. It's time to start talking, ladies! Talk this monster out of our lives! Talk this monster down!

---

1. <u>Evidence Against the Views of the Abolitionists, Consisting of Physical and Moral Proofs, of the Natural Inferiority of the Negroes</u>, Richard H. Colfax, (New York: James T.M. Bleakley), 1833, p.16.

2. <u>New Physiognomy, or Signs of Character as manifested Through Temperament and External Forms and Especially in "the human face divine."</u>, Samuel R. Wells, (New York: Fowler and Wells), 1866. All images and text relating to phrenology and physiognomy in this chapter taken from this edition.

Chapter 5
WE DO IT FOR THEIR LOVE

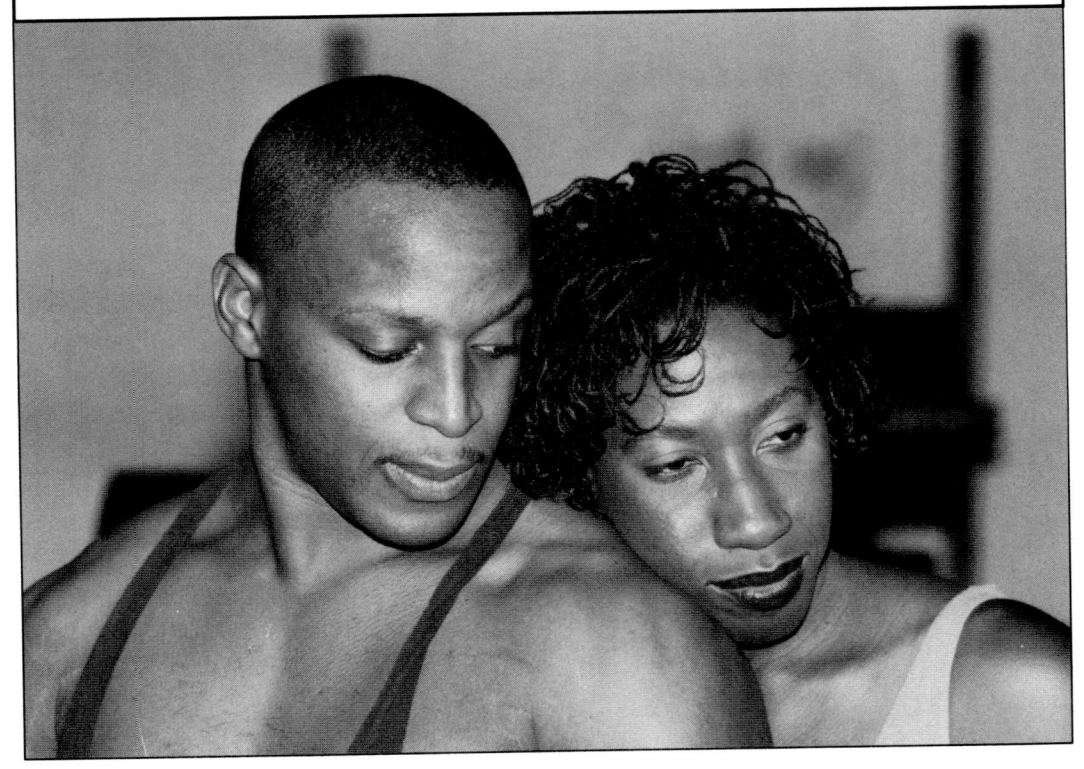

Though African American men and women have made great strides working side by side through the decades in the struggle for equal rights, we still have real problems dealing with each other on a personal level. This is no secret. A lot of attention has been paid to the disfunctionality of black male/female relationships and the various sources of stress on our men and women. Stress has been linked to things like high unemployment and dangerous social conditions, and the impact of these on the ability of men and women to sustain healthy, stable relationships.

While I agree with much of what has been set forth, I do not feel that the reasons for our problems are solely external in nature. Our history has shown that negative social and economic conditions do not necessarily mean <u>weak</u> relationships. Recently, we've also seen that positive conditions resulting in greater upward mobility, do not necessarily lead to <u>strong</u> relationships.

Psychologists would agree that low self-esteem is something that can be both the result, and the root cause of the other sources of stress that undeniably make relationships difficult to sustain. Unfortunately, we often use the expression, "low self-esteem" rather carelessly. We think we know what this means, but we rarely discuss where it comes from, except to blame external factors like poverty and the lack of role models. We <u>have</u> role models. We've always had them, even in the worst of times. But what is it about us that prevents so many of us from internalizing and acting on their positive examples?

Studying this 'hair thing' has made me look closely into the question of self-esteem and relationships. The way we feel about our appearance has to have a profound impact on our ability to form healthy, significant relationships. Over and over again, I've asked myself, "Why do we so dislike our natural hair?" Some of the answers come from looking into our history. The most important answers however, are to be found by taking a close look at the ways we have **internalized** that history.

This is an important distinction. What has that history made of us? *What have we become, when statistics demonstrate that our men are abandoning our women on a mass scale? What have we become,*

> *The way we feel about our appearance has to have a profound impact on our ability to form healthy, significant relationships.*

> *To a greater or lesser degree, we have lost our ability to see, believe in, and be empowered by the physical beauty that is unique to our own kind.*

when the physical traits of our women are acceptable objects of ridicule in our culture? What have we become, when our women feel that covering up or correcting nature is the only way to make themselves lovable, or even acceptable, both to men and to other women?

I have come up with a term for our dilemma: As African Americans, we are in the throes of what I call an 'aesthetic crisis.' To a greater or lesser degree, we have lost our ability to see, believe in, and be empowered by the physical beauty that is unique to our own kind. This, as much as anything else, affects our ability to cherish one another in relationships.

Speaking from experience, this loss sets in fairly early. Young Black girls in this society, trying to figure out how to be attractive, are up against tremendous odds. I have several friends today who, despite their African cultural orientation, have daughters at that age where their natural hair is no longer acceptable to them. Sometimes braided extensions help them through the crisis, but at other times they resort to the harshest chemical extremes. Peer pressure to look acceptable, meaning like everyone else around them, can be stronger than the best family values. Ironically, the same hair issues come up for our girls whether they are in environments that are predominantly African American or not.

I have given a lot of thought to my own grooming choices over the years, and the ways I have devised to be perceived as normal and acceptable. As a younger woman, like most of my peers, I had no idea whose truth I was running after. For this reason, my quest for male attention often had a desperate, hopeless feeling to it. I was always sensitive to the way I believed men were reacting to my physical appearance. That was especially true of my hair. Like most of us, I went to incredible lengths over the years to get their attention. I just had to have that illusive 'right look', meaning of course

> *I just had to have that illusive 'right look', meaning of course the no-naps-in-sight, swoosh-when-you-turn-your-head-to-look*

the no-naps-in-sight, swoosh-when-you-turn-your-head-to-look look.

I have tried the lye and the glycerin, the extensions and all of 'their' products that promised to make my hair long and silky. These products never delivered, but I would try anything that promised to give that delayed bounce action when I flipped my head around in the sexy, Hollywood way we all rehearsed when we were girls with half-slips or tee shirts on our heads. This was the look that was sure to get the man. I confess, I did it for their love. Little did I know at the time, but because the men didn't know either whose truth they were running after, they were, for the most part, incapable - not unwilling, but incapable - of giving it.

This is the essence of our aesthetic crisis. Although it is related to other external factors, I believe it has more to do with how we experience two things in our lives that are basic to all human beings. These are **Beauty** and **Truth**. Our experience of these two forces affects us throughout our lives on a very deep level. As humans, we have a strong natural urge to connect the two, but as African Americans, too often in our daily lives, Beauty is not related to what is True for us at all. This disconnection is a very profound one and it plays an important role in how we structure our choices and responses to the conditions around us. I believe that it is a critical factor in the success of black male/female relationships, as well as black family relationships.

Ensuring the convergence of Beauty and Truth is one of our culture's most important tasks, because this creates an empowering sense of certainty for us. Our ability to cause Beauty and Truth ideals to converge is one of our most profound human resources. Literally, it is one of those higher functions that set us apart as a species from the animal world. We make use of it to structure, evaluate and celebrate our world. Beneath it all, the Beauty/Truth connection is really what people fight for, sacrifice for and defend.

When this connection is intact,

it can produce a value system that supports a feeling of healthy integration within the community and society as a whole. On the other hand, if for some reason this connection is impaired, there can remain little to fight for, sacrifice for or defend. Our lives, our goals, our very bodies may even begin to seem pointless, worthless or even ridiculous. Psychologists will tell you that this is no exaggeration!

You must be familiar with the extension/weave jokes that are so widely popular among African American comedians these days. Although joking insults about black women's hair go back many decades, it used to be that our men made fun of us if our hair was too 'nappy.' The content of the jokes has changed, but their negative message has not. Just as we may expect, it's damned if you do and damned if you don't when it comes to our hair. I wonder how funny our quest for long, straight hair would seem to our men if all of a sudden **they** were expected to wear their hair longer too, in order to conform to acceptable standards of appearance. Would they be able to resist the pressure and show more cultural fortitude than we have?

> *I wonder how funny our quest for long, straight hair would seem to our men if all of a sudden they were expected to wear their hair longer too, in order to conform to acceptable standards of appearance. Do you think they would not be re-inventing "Conk" faster than you could blink an eye?*

I don't think so! Do you think they would not be re-inventing "Conk" faster than you could blink an eye?

The fact that so many of our men still find it acceptable for even a few among them to bash and scapegoat on our women's chronic beauty dilemmas displays an alarming lack of empathy. I have to ask "Who are they identifying with?" if not us and our efforts over the past decades to neutralize those same awful stereotypes about our race that they have had to deal with. Our successes are also their successes and our failures are theirs as well. Could we get a little help here, guys?

These male 'jokers' in my view suffer to an alarming degree from the aesthetic crisis I mention earlier. The resulting practice of self-deception allows them to make light of the solutions we women have come up with for our hair. They would have the world believe that women alone are the ones with the problems, when they are just as hung-up a we are. We are trying to get their attention, but since they are as confused as we are about the necessary connection between Beauty and Truth, it's really tough to second-guess what they are **capable** of seeing as beautiful in us!

I need to explain what I mean by "the necessary connection between Beauty and Truth." Don't be misled by the common usage of these terms. We may think that beauty just deals with the superficial level of things, but nothing could be further from the truth! Beauty also applies to ideas and ideologies, as well as feelings, actions and intentions of all kinds. The superficial features of a person or an object become markers (or symbols) for what we feel is housed at the deeper levels. These superficial attributes (hair, skin, etc.) have no value whatsoever <u>unless</u> they are linked to these deeper level truths.

The link between appearance and our deeply felt values may be very subtle, but in fact we are constantly making judgments about everything that comes into our experience. When we decide that something is Beautiful (meaning 'pleasing', 'right', or even 'appropriate'), you can bet that we have determined on a deep level that it also stands in a proper relationship to what we believe is True (meaning 'accurate,' 'natural,' 'virtuous,' or 'intended' by a creator we believe in).

Most of us have no real need to think much about beauty and truth in the way that I am describing. In fact, it is precisely the role of someones

> *We may think that beauty just deals with the superficial level of things, but nothing could be further from the truth!*

culture to make it **unnecessary** for them to have to justify why they feel right about their world. To the individual who is culturally integrated, truth and beauty become mutually supportive concepts that reinforce customary thinking. If a person has always felt validated by society, whatever is perceived as beauty is also seen as true, and truth is intuitively experienced as beautiful. Living in a world with this kind of integrity gives them ready access to empowering and motivating creative energies.

What I am suggesting is that in contrast to this ideal scenario, African Americans as a cultural group have lost the ability to define beauty as truth for ourselves. This loss has resulted in a widespread lack of confidence in the ways we structure, evaluate and celebrate our world.

In extreme cases, rather than feeling empowered, motivated and creatively enriched by our involvement with our own kind, we may feel inhibited or even angry at our own folks without really knowing why. In our confusion and sense of powerlessness, we may react with aversion to people like us. This is really an expression of fear or disgust at those unnamed, misunderstood parts of ourselves. Expressions of anger on the one hand, and impulses toward self-denigrating behavior on the other, define the range of responses left open to someone like this, as they try to either survive the odds of a struggle they don't really understand, or simply jump their sinking cultural ship! I believe that the chronic beauty dilemmas of our women are a visible symptom of this deep cultural confusion.

When extreme attitudes emerge, they are certainly, at least in part, holdovers from the past when our social ways and physical characteristics were taken as concrete proof that we were culture-less beings, and therefore an inferior race of people. Ironically, in another place and time, our languages, our dress, our features, skin color and hair had once confirmed for us in an unambiguous way that we were the True sons and daughters of life. Centuries of cultural domination however, placed serious stress on our normal ways of understanding the empowering truth and beauty of our being and ways of living. We were left swimming in a confusing cultural soup, and we are only just now learning how to sift out and re-evaluate our own essence in

> *They (men) might be polite to you if you don't have 'the look', but they will crawl for you if you do!*

order to better savor its importance in relation to the whole.

Most black women I know are intelligent, sensitive people. An alarming number of us however, have problems on some level with black men as a group. When we try to talk this out among ourselves, several issues come up as being responsible for the rift that undeniably exists: Depressed communities; the stress of underemployment; large scale incarceration of our men; even upward mobility leading to cultural abandonment; and of course, the always menacing curse of the 'white woman.' Many of our women have given over to feelings of powerlessness when it comes to healing the relationships with our men. We are enraged at being treated as though **what** we are necessarily sets limits on the quality of relationships we can have.

What we really want is for our men to acknowledge the beauty within us, and for this acknowledgment to lead to real, honest engagement in our lives together. What we too often get, when we are not being ridiculed, is indifference or neglect. Men's attitudes about our hair are most often revealed, not in what they say but in how they behave, or in most cases, their lack of committed response.

In fact, no matter what he may really be feeling, the average male in my experience will either understate his opinion about a black woman's hair, or say nothing at all. I interpret a refusal to comment as a form of comment, that usually means "Your hair is your issue, not mine!" (OK, so maybe they don't want to get their a---- chewed off by saying the wrong thing, either.) In any case, before Sisterlocks, I had rarely seen men moved to making unsolicited compliments about how stunning a black woman's hair looked. I would even wager that the vast majority of our women have never gotten consistently enthusiastic reactions to their hair from their men.

There is one clear exception to this rule, of course. Just make it look like 'theirs,' ladies, and you will move men to spontaneous adoration! Today there are more and more advanced, supposedly 'natural' chemical formulas that will help you accomplish this miracle. Make it long and straight, give it bounce, make it sway the way a woman's hair is supposed to, and you will create a man-magnet! Our men fantasize about these things, you know. They crave seeing a woman's hair blowing in the wind. Their fingers itch for tresses to run through. They might be polite to you if you don't have 'the look,' but they will crawl for you if you do!

I'm exaggerating. But only just a little. Many women who have gone from Afro to 'free-flow' can attest to the increased attention they get from men. Our men may not openly admit it, but most will pass up the Afro for the weave every time. But are we really surprised, ladies, to find them running after the same illusion that we are running after, and for the same reasons?

Despite all of the frustrations, we continue to try to find ways to attract their attention, knowing instinctively that physical attraction is an immutable lure. However, we are caught in a sort of "Catch 22" because in order for our physical beauty to have meaning and value for our intended ones, it must be rooted on some level in that person's sense of what is true. But what if that person's sense of truth is distorted?

Most of us are aware that the beauty standards in this country were not created by us or for us, and that this whole 'hair thing' is related to the fact that, without feeling we have much choice, we are upholding the very standards that negate our own natural characteristics. Under these conditions for example, our natural hair **cannot** be truly beautiful. Knowing this, we continue nonetheless to adorn ourselves in ways we think will hold the attention and admiration of our men. This includes not only our husbands and lovers, but also our sons and fathers, and our male extended family and community members.

People may talk about the irony of our behavior; they may joke and complain about it, but after all is said and done, most of us continue in our same old ways. How is it we can identify this as a problem, all agree that it is unfortunate - even tragic - and still go back time and again to ways that are hopelessly self-negating?

Part of the answer lies in our anxiety about abandoning the majority standards of beauty - even though they may be false for us - because doing this may alienate us further from our men ... and you know, this anxiety is justified. Our men suffer just as deeply as we do from the confusion resulting from our inability to create a conjunction between Beauty and Truth in our daily lives. I would be willing to bet that most of us - male and female - feel as uncomfortable about natural hair as we do about some of the extreme chemical processes we use. Nonetheless, most of us have at one time or another tried to make our hair into what we told ourselves was beautiful, all the while knowing deep down that it was not.

Because we are so utterly unfamiliar with our natural hair, it carries a very low truth value for us, compared to the value assigned to straight hair. So we are left with being 'damned' on the one hand for embracing a standard that has a high truth value but is false for us, and 'damned' on the other hand if we embrace a standard that may be true for us but is under-valued by the majority of those around us!

For me, this illustrates the utter triumph of the racialist view we have existed under as a culture. A clear sign that this view has triumphed is seen in how the victim continues to behave in a way that replicates racist behavior against itself. It may be puzzling to some how this can continue to be such a compelling problem for African Americans as a group when so many of the outward structures of our racially-based society have been demolished or reformed. Laws have been changed; far-reaching social programs have been enacted for the betterment of our communities; economic barriers have eroded significantly. The fact is that we have worked on these <u>outward</u> issues much more aggressively than on those that involve repairing our wounded cultural psyche.

The brand of racist oppression practiced during the era of slavery inflicted wounds that cut much deeper than the social, political or economic levels. An indication of this is to be found in the fact that whether African Americans are rich or poor, whether we live in cities or towns, slums or mansions, whether we are democrats or republicans, we all tend to harbor the same types of negative feelings and anxieties about ourselves as a group, and specifically about our hair.

Because of this, no social, political or economic remedies <u>alone</u> will get to the bottom of what we feel is wrong with us, or why we have such

> *Since the wounds of racism have affected us at the deepest level of our basic humanity, we have to look for remedies on that level.*

a problem with each other. Since the wounds of racism have affected us at the deepest level of our basic humanity, we have to look for remedies on that level. This must be done if we are to complete the healing process begun by political and social activists. It is now up to us to look inside, identify and repair the disconnection resulting from our historical experience.

On the most basic level then, when we look at relationships between men and women, we have to ask what attracts us to one another. As much as we might want to believe that we are supposed to look at the quality of the inner person - and we should, of course - we cannot deny that there is a basic part of our make-up that either feels physically attracted or not. It is wrong to downplay or negate physical attraction because it is <u>always</u> a factor, whether we acknowledge it or not. At times, our actions appear to be driven purely by our hormones, but, unless we are mentally defective, there is <u>always</u> some judgment involved. In a way, the animals are the lucky ones because they have their instincts to rely on through the relationship process. There is no real judgment involved in their choice of partners, at least not in the true sense of the word. On the other hand, humans rely very heavily on judgment. This judgment is often so deeply conditioned that it is unconscious. This is where culture comes in. Where animals have **instinct,** we have **truth value** as determined by our culture. So, where an animal knows that it has found the right mate through instinct, we rely on a feeling that the outward traits we are attracted to have a high truth value for us. When an acceptable truth value is reached, we feel right with our choices.

What I am describing here can be thought of as a basic pattern of human attraction. For African Americans however, this pattern has been significantly distorted, since the truth values we assign cannot be relied upon. This situation can cause a deep sense of confusion and emotional dissatisfaction.

Most of us may not be consciously aware of this, living as we do in a society where the idea of individual choice is so highly valued. We can easily tell ourselves that the ways we make ourselves look are simply voluntary, and based on some independent personal code. So when a woman says that she always wears her hair straightened simply because she likes it that way, she truly may not be aware that she is really skating on the surface of a very deep human tragedy that she is involved in perpetuating. Or when a man pleads with his female partner not to cut her chemically altered hair in order to go natural, he may not realize the degree to which he may be helping to make her unlovable.

We operate today at the tip of a tremendously deep iceberg that started forming a long time ago. The part that remains beneath the surface is not visible, but still determines the conscious choices floating on the surface. When we are unaware of what is beneath the surface, self-negation can feel like the truth!

I used to think that men had it easy when it came to hair, and we women had all the hang-ups. Today I am convinced that this 'hair thing' is not just a woman thing. Men, too have hang-ups about their hair types, the dominant preference being of course straight or wavy over kinky. Once I realized this, I couldn't figure out how some men could get away with being so judgmental about women's hair, and others at the other extreme could act as though they were totally unaware of the problem. We see this in both their words and their actions, from the insults and jokes on the one hand, to passive-aggressive neglect of women because of their looks, on the other. At both extremes, these negative behaviors are sometimes pushed to the point of cruelty. This is really troubling because when the men in a group can so easily turn their own women into objects of ridicule or

> *I used to think that men had it easy when it came to hair, and we women had all the hang-ups.*

scorn, or relegate them to a status of non-importance, it is an indication of their own thinly camouflaged self-hatred.

Part of our dilemma is really quite obvious: We're Americans, and for more and more of us, **that's not all bad!** We have been raised on TV and Hollywood, just like the majority of Americans. Though many of us continue to think of ourselves as an isolated sub-group, statistically that is not true any longer. We are internalizing their codes, and they are internalizing ours. We have sung along with Mitch, left it to Beaver and dreamt of Jeannie. We have spun the Wheel of Fortune, and some of us even won! We have grown up not just cursing, but also celebrating 'their' images, and this has had a profound effect on us as a culture. It has made us much less predictable and much more complex. Should we be surprised then, that our men are conditioned to look for the Bo or the Vanna in us? (Dismayed perhaps, but not surprised.)

We all have been subjected to a life-long conditioning process that teaches what is 'normal' and acceptable in our society, and to some degree, we all aspire to these things. **Normalcy after all is the pre-condition to beauty.** Our greatest task today is to ensure that our true images get included in what is considered normal. With things as they are now, this culture says that women are most acceptable when their non-African traits are dominant. We African American women spend our lives trying to acquire and keep these traits.

The tragedy is that our willingness to sacrifice the basic truth value of our natural expressions of beauty profoundly wounds our humanity. By relinquishing the deep and necessary connection between truth and beauty, we not only lay ourselves open to the ridicule of those who pick up on our lack of connectedness, but worse, we actually <u>feel</u> ridiculous within ourselves. And here I am perfectly serious; this is not exaggeration.

Ask yourself what is truly beautiful hair to the average African

Ask yourself what is truly beautiful hair to the average African American man in your experience?

American man in your experience? There may be several answers to that question, but how often do you see a convergence in his mind, between beauty and African-textured hair? This is what has to change, both for our men, and especially for ourselves. The growing number of women who have chosen to allow their natural hair to express itself, often do so in spite of their men, not because of them. And more power to them!

Mark my words, as more of us restore our own Beauty/Truth connection within and create a new reality for ourselves, more of our men will wish to share in that fuller cultural experience. This is a task that falls on us to initiate. Women who have restored that connection find they are left with exactly what they deserve - men in their lives who are capable of seeing, appreciating, reveling in and loving the truth of their natural beauty!

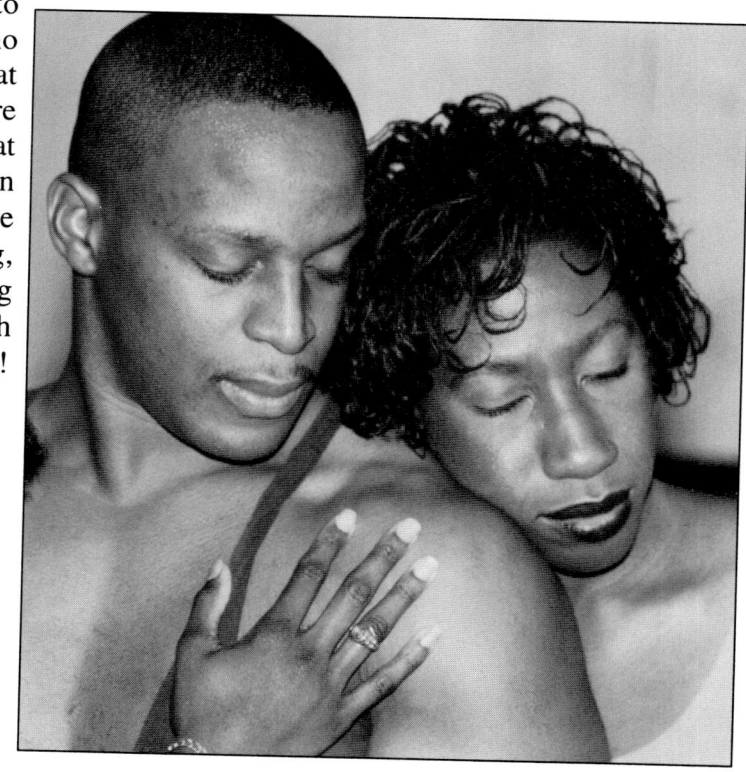

PART TWO

The Sisterlocks Approach

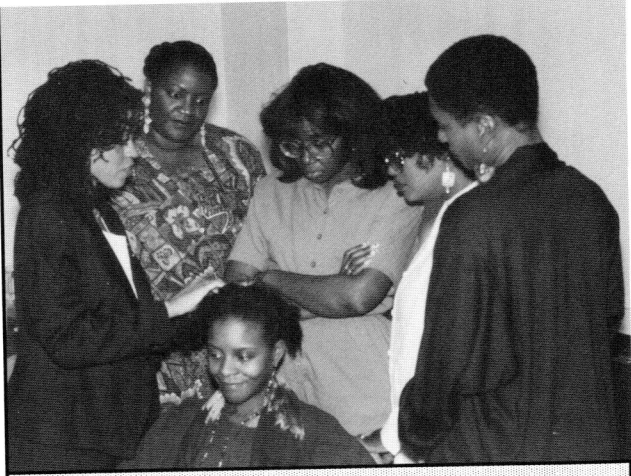

You've read the previous section, and now you understand why hair can be a very powerful symbol in our lives. It has been a negative preoccupation for me from a very young age, and I don't think I'm much different from most African American women. In fact, every serious conversation I've ever had on this topic confirmed that our hair issues shape our lives in more ways than we openly admit.

How do our women live with the fact that our natural hair type is considered a handicap? It is no secret that many of us feel helpless to change what feels like an unfortunate fact life. But a growing number are choosing to go against the grain and explore the range of natural hair alternatives. The number of natural options is growing daily too, as more hair care specialists are becoming skilled in natural methods, and popular demand is growing. Women who choose natural alternatives are discovering a new way of feeling about themselves. The transition doesn't always come easily, but the rewards usually surpass all expectations.

The Sisterlocks Approach offers one way for women to experience their natural hair. It is not an anti-straight-hair approach, it is a pro-natural-hair approach. I say this because Sisterlocks is based on a philosophy that acknowledges our difficult past, respects the transformation we must make at present, and offers spectacular natural solutions on which to build our future.

Here are 3 ideas at the heart of the Sisterlocks Approach:

1. Our hair dilemmas are not exactly about hair.
2. Until natural methods are prominent among our hair care choices, hair straightening and hair processing will continue to carry the unfortunate stigma of the 'cover-up.'
3. The value we place on hair is not a given; it is determined by the prevailing norms of our culture.

With an understanding of the ideas covered in Part One, you will certainly appreciate the following insights about the Sisterlocks solution.

Chapter 6
JUST ANOTHER HAIR CARE REVOLUTION

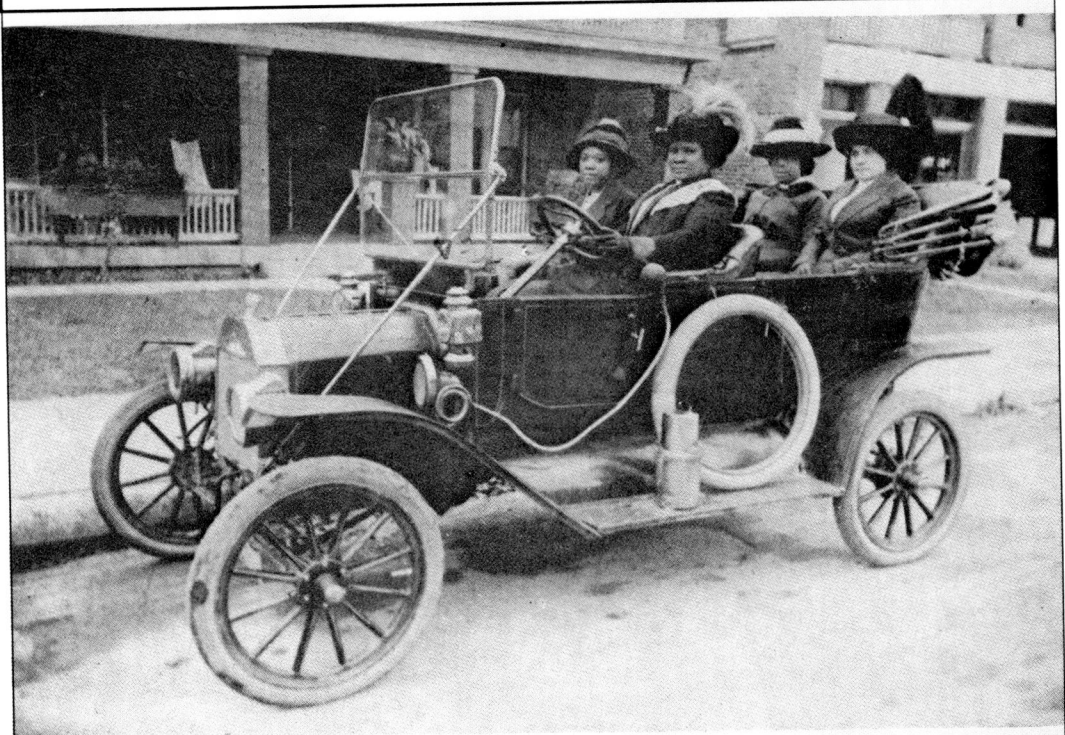

"I am a woman who came from the cotton fields of the South. I was promoted from there to the washtub. Then I was promoted to the cook kitchen, and from there I PROMOTED MYSELF into the business of manufacturing hair goods and preparations... I have built my own factory on my own ground."

Speaking at the National Negro Business League, 1912 Convention

Madam C.J. Walker

> *Her approach was hugely popular, and her legions of employees earned salaries many times greater than the average for white males.*

I have long been familiar with the accomplishments of Madame C.J. Walker. No "Who's Who" list in the area of black hair care would be complete without this remarkable woman whose accomplishments included being the first black millionairess, perfecting the hair straightening comb, and helping to professionalize the black hair care industry. Surely, we've all seen the signature photographs of her flaunting that grand style of hers. She was a self-made woman, whose success stood for all of us - her accomplishments were our accomplishments.

Her ascension to greatness has been thoroughly documented. "Madame Walker's Wonderful Hair Grower" was one of her original products. It developed out of her search for a remedy for her own damaged hair. She began her business by marketing it door to door. She also developed a design for the straightening comb that made it practical for use in African-type hair. She established a manufacturing concern for the production of her products and tools, and employed scores of African Americans in the process. She developed a professional training program that resulted in salons and schools nationwide. These produced over 25,000 "beauty culturists" dedicated to the beauty concerns of black women. This was all done before there were any boards of cosmetology with externally imposed or inappropriate guidelines for how to address the grooming concerns of black women.

Her approach was hugely popular, and her legions of employees earned salaries many times greater than the average for white males. In short she, along with a handful of her contemporaries, created an industry from the ground up based on their ability to recognize a demand and adequately supply the needs of black women. Walker took an approach to hair care and grooming that was right for the women of her day, and they supported her efforts on a mass scale. This was a hair care revolution of sorts that moved our women ahead in their efforts to create more opportunities for themselves within the mainstream.

What is happening today in the natural hair care industry feels in many ways like the latest phase of that hair care revolution launched at the century's dawning. We seem to be coming full circle in terms of many of the issues Mme. Walker stood for. Where our foremothers' task was to forge pathways over uncharted, openly hostile cultural terrain, ours is to develop and expand opportunities in areas where the barriers have largely been broken down by those who went before. Ironically, our foremothers used the weapon of conformity in their physical appearance to challenge their systematic exclusion from the mainstream.. Today, it is our challenge to move forward by asserting and openly celebrating our uniqueness. Now, as was the case nearly a century ago, there is a ground swell movement growing in support of our new mission. More and more of our women are saying **YES** to their glorious uniqueness, and are demanding acceptance, both inside and outside of the home.

As a result of this, our hair care professionals are feeling pressure to respond to the changing demands of our women. Their actual response to date however, has been painfully slow. Imagine that with the 21st century upon us, most of our women who want to explore natural options in hair styling still have no place to go, except in most cases, underground. Have you ever asked yourself why it is that the vast majority of braiders and natural hair care practitioners find themselves in situations where they can not open public, legitimate businesses without being threatened with fines and shop closures? Like Mme. C.J. Walker, they are responding appropriately to a growing demand among our women, only this time the demand is for a more culturally unique approach to beauty than can be found in most mainstream salons.

Like Mme. Walker and her followers, the present day natural hair practitioners have developed a whole new array of approaches to hair care,

> *Like Mme. Walker and her followers, the present day natural hair practitioners have developed a whole new array of approaches to hair care, specifically suited to our hair types and lifestyles.*

specifically suited to our hair types and lifestyles. What is it that allowed Walker and her associates to become hugely successful at the turn of the last century, while her counterparts at the turn of this century remain relegated to kitchens, dens and salons without addresses? The biggest obstacle to the growth of the natural hair care industry is plainly clear to those of us who are in the trenches of this revolution: Inappropriate government regulations. These regulations define and defend an approach to hair care that was never designed with black people in mind, and therefore gives little or no consideration to our natural hair types. Nonetheless, this narrow and often harmful approach is projected as universally relevant. So, with the force of the law behind them, boards of cosmetology nationwide effectively outlaw any approaches that deviate from their own, even - as in the case of braiding and natural hair care - when these so-called deviant practices are necessary to the well being of our hair types and represent appropriate responses to massive demand.

Plainly stated, the ability of our own professionals to respond to the needs of our own women is being hampered by the way the cosmetology industry is set up. They have the legal right to set limits on what we do, although they lack even the most basic sensitivity to it or understanding of it. As long as it deals with hair, they say, you will do it our way! So, while Mme. C.J. Walker could see a need and fill it, beauty care specialists today are forced to abide by regulations that are inherently in opposition to practices essential to the healthy hair care needs of those with naturally textured hair.

Let me be even more specific. No matter where

you go in this modern world, (and I have been an extensive world traveler for many years) you see the same embarrassing scenario: *Women with African-type hair have the worst cared for hair on the planet! Our hair is dry, broken off, won't grow, burned off, falling out, weak and tired! You know I'm not lying. It is the single most humiliating source of cultural embarrassment we know. "Black Women Don't Have No Hair!"* This lie looks like the truth because the so-called legitimate approach to hair care - the only one that is legally open to us - is ruining our hair!

No wonder we have such deep feelings of inferiority and shame about it! So many of us live with that gut feeling that there is something very wrong with having tightly textured hair, and with this as our reality, we never allow ourselves the freedom to even consider a natural hair style.

I don't think it's putting too fine a point on this to say that this 'hair thing' has literally brought us to our knees! And this is not because our hair care professionals who have been trained in the mainstream system are incompetent. They, for the most part, have been 'appropriately' trained, but by the very system of cosmetology that I am now challenging. That is exactly the problem! The approach to hair care taught by traditional cosmetology is in some respects, just plain WRONG for African-type hair! Despite the myths that we have bought into for generations, our hair is NOT at its best when it is chemicalized and otherwise stressed to conform to the straight hair standards that are imposed

Despite the myths that we have bought into for generations, our hair is NOT at its best when it is chemicalized and otherwise stressed to conform to the straight hair standards that are imposed on us.

on us.

The cosmetology industry for the most part refuses to recognize the legitimacy of the work of our own experts, who have developed approaches to hair care uniquely suited to our hair types. The approaches I refer to include not just specific hair braiding and locking, shampooing and ongoing maintenance techniques, but also alternative approaches to salon (or environment) management and the delivery of customer and business services. For example, I find that with my Sisterlocks system, where the initial locking session takes me from 7 to 10 hours to complete, my customers are more comfortable in a home-like setting where they can enjoy relative privacy, snooze, read, watch a movie or listen to music. Having this type of customer sit for such an extended length of time in a traditional salon setting designed for procedures taking no more than 2-3 hours, seems to me to raise a health and safety concern. A customer's physical comfort has to be at least as important as the technician's need for clean hands and clean tools.

Our experts routinely achieve attractive, versatile styles that are stress-free on the hair and promote hair growth. Our approach to hair care however, would **never** have developed within the existing cosmetology structure. I would also say that the salon setting itself as we know it is not particularly conducive to the success of a natural hair care enterprise. Nevertheless, prevailing laws continue to impose inappropriate training and licensing requirements on our natural hair care specialists. This is true despite the fact that cosmetology schools cannot teach the braiders and locticians the skills they will need when applying their trade in the natural hair care world.

Madame Walker appeared not to have been confronted with legal restrictions of this kind as she worked to establish black hair care as a viable industry in the early 1900s. This may have been owing more to a lack of sophistication among law makers than to a feeling of generosity on the part of the then city fathers. Fortunately for her, the onslaught unleashed upon those who followed her example, did not come until after her death. The history of both the cosmetology boards in this country, and the barbering boards that preceded them, is littered with examples of exclusionary practices based on either race or gender.

For example, though early barbering boards would ignore the activities of African American barbers working in their homes, these barbers could be cited if they dared to open public establishments. Not surprisingly, African American barbers of that era were often self-taught, or trained within structures not recognized or credited by the mainstream. This was either because the training schools would not admit blacks, or because they could not receive appropriate training in cutting and grooming black hair in those schools.

In the same vein, when women sought to enter the mainstream as hair culturists, they were met with opposition from the all-male barbering trade. That struggle ended in the formation of a new, independent board of cosmetology, which ironically, now seeks to negate the validity of our natural hair care industry.

Timing is everything, and these new boards were forming at a time when the budding black hair culturalist industry was establishing itself in major cities throughout the country. The refined straightening comb designs and specialized hair care products of Mme. Walker, Annie Turnbo Malone and Sarah Spencer Washington were

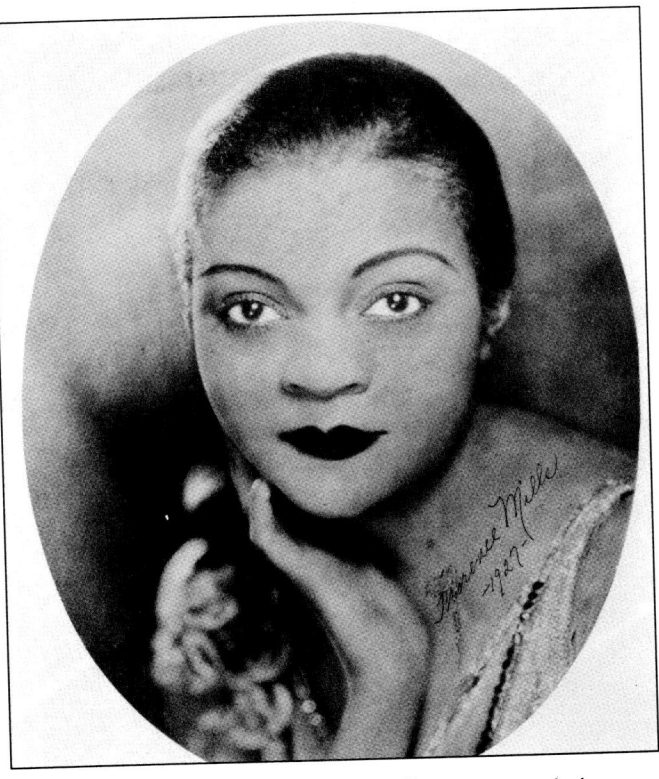

Performing idols like Florence Mills set new straight-hair beauty standards for African American women during the early decades of the 20th century.

setting the standard for black hair care. This was a time when hair straightening was fast becoming the norm for the progressive black woman.

Clearly, hair care practices at that time reflected Black women's dire need for social conformity, over and above the concrete needs of our unique hair type. Because of this fact, on the surface, the standard cosmetology approach that was being formalized nationwide, did not seem to go against our own ways of thinking. The fact is that this newly refined practice of hair straightening (along with skin lightning which was also becoming widely practiced) was hotly debated within black communities, and in the black press across the nation. Individuals challenged Mme. Walker and others for encouraging our women to deny themselves in their pursuit of acceptability in the form of Caucasian physical attributes. It is ironic that despite their individual success and empowering of so many others, the innovations brought about by those like Mme. Walker played an unwitting role in the erasure of African American uniqueness at this crucial time.

As standards within the cosmetology industry became set, the law of conformity became the official law of the land in hair care for African Americans. These standards remained in force until the early 60's when, following on the cultural nationalist or "Black Power" movement, short and medium natural styles exploded onto the scene. This took large numbers of black hair dressers by surprise. They were totally unprepared to groom, and dress black hair without first altering its texture through chemicals or heat straightening.

Ironically, rather than taking up the banner of this second phase of our hair care revolution to help professionalize it and perfect techniques, the majority of cosmetologists and shop owners simply felt their businesses were being threatened, and reacted as such. They believed that women (and men) with Afros would no longer need their hair straightening services, and so, would no longer need <u>them</u>. Their lack of vision prevented them from imagining any other services they might offer.

The 'natural' was viewed as a stepchild at best; a fad to be tolerated. A few traditionally trained hair care professionals responded differently however, notably Mr. William Morrow, who popularized the "Afro Comb", and marketed his services internationally as a consultant on how to cut and style natural, African-type hair. Despite the more progressive efforts of Morrow and others, the mainstream approach to correcting black hair for the most part, did not adapt itself to the growing demands for natural hair and ethnic braids. This refusal of the present cosmetology industry to become more inclusive of ethnic hair care during this time, marked the birth of the renegade natural hair care industry.

This is the time when, along with the Afro, the braiding and hair locking arts began to make their appearance. Though fairly widespread today, what some refer to as 'ethnic hair styling' involved a radical departure from the mainstream cosmetology approach to hair care. Today, braids are widely worn in all of our major cities. Many varieties of natural locks and twists are becoming equally popular, and it is the 'hair renegades' who are responsible for this. Although some of these renegades have chosen to acquire cosmetology licenses, the majority of them do not see any practical relevance in becoming cosmetologists.

Given this fact, we have to ask where braiders and locticians go, if not to cosmetology schools, to learn their arts? Also, how can a person who wants to try braids or a natural 'do, be sure about choosing a

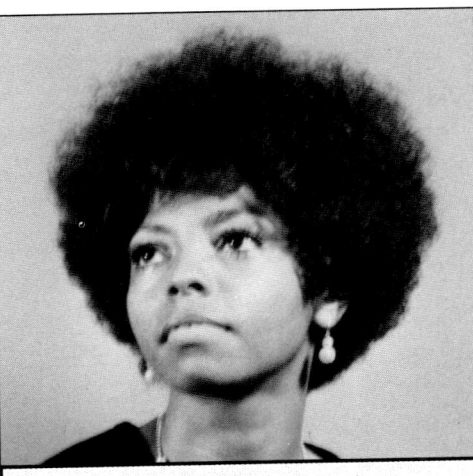

> *The 'natural' was viewed as a stepchild at best; a fad to be tolerated. This refusal of the cosmetology industry to become more inclusive ... marked the birth of the renegade natural hair care industry.*

practitioner who has been properly trained? These questions point to the current dilemma within the natural hair care industry. The problem is not simply that the existing cosmetology structure is inappropriate, but that its legal monopoly prevents any alternative structure from emerging. Clearly, this monopoly must end, and Sisterlocks, along with other braiding and natural hair care specialists and associations, is working very hard to bring this about.

Sisterlocks has created one alternative to the cosmetology approach. This system brings together several areas of specialization and concern, and enjoys a nation-wide track record for delivering a quality alternative to chemical services. The system involves a range of trademarked services, from a salon

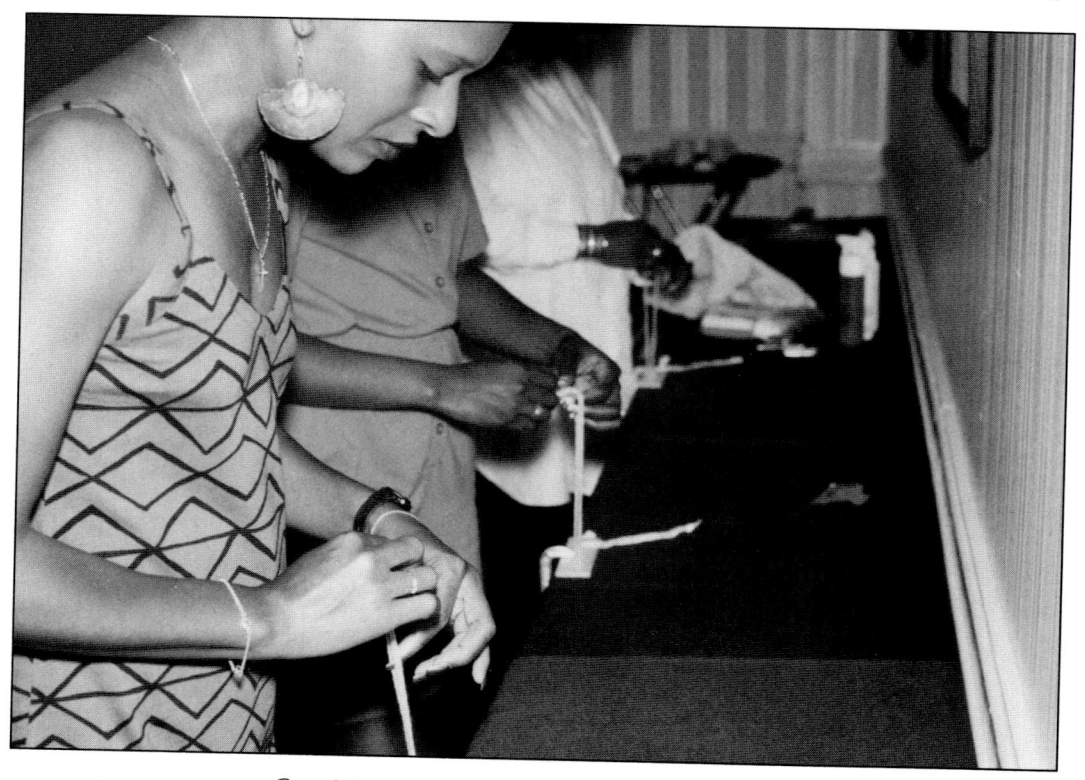

Sisterlocks trainees practice techniques on practice boards.

concept to training courses and videos and even a product line. It also involves a private certification program designed to provide customers with an assurance of quality. All of our training is fully standardized so that a Certified Consultant in Miami, Florida is able to do the same brand-name quality job as a Consultant in Anaheim, California.

Our curriculum is lengthy compared to most approaches to teaching a natural hair technique. We stress not just technique, but also an understanding of our unique hair structure, and we focus on long term care of the natural locks. What does all this mean in practical terms? It means that since we are a trademark company, no one can legally claim to offer Sisterlocks salon services, training or products unless they are really giving customers the genuine article. For the client, it helps take the guess work out of finding a competent practitioner without risking the health of the hair. Potential clients can simply phone the home office to find out if a person in their area has been properly trained, or authorized to train others or distribute our products. This approach also works well in helping to insure quality performance by our consultants. Satisfied customers let us know which of our Consultants are giving good service. Dissatisfied customers let us know which of our Consultants may need additional tips or training, or in extreme cases, need to have their status revoked.

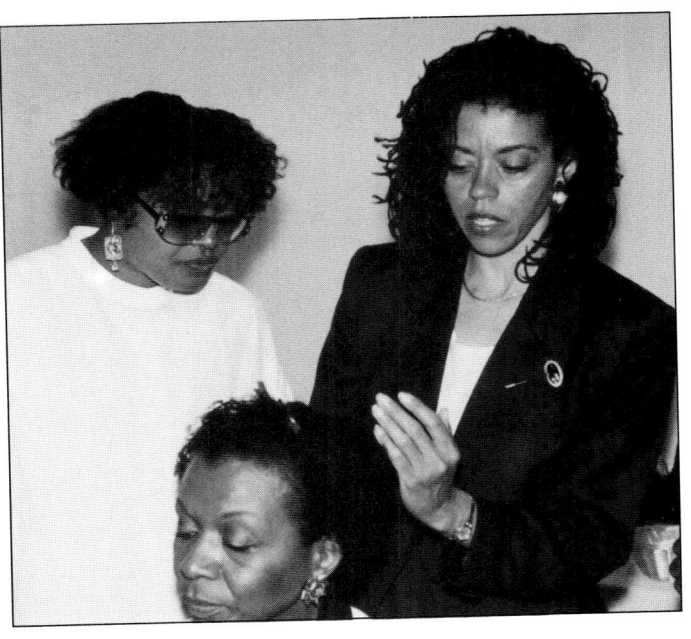

Sisterlocks is a unique, natural hair care system that is responding to the needs of millions of women. This system evolved out of a combination of my technical expertise in hair arrangement, my ability to successfully analyze and resolve issues relating to our uniquely structured hair type (not taught in any cosmetology school I know of), my academic expertise in curriculum (training) development, and an entrepreneurial spirit that I consider to be a legacy from my female forebearers. The structure of my business takes advantage of the fully legal options available to entrepreneurs of every description throughout this land. **What purpose could possibly be served by making this approach illegal?**

Back in 1992 I was the only person in the world with Sisterlocks, but even then I knew I had come upon something that had the potential for radically changing the way women like me related to ourselves as women in the world. That realization brought with it a sense of elation that can scarcely be described. At the same time I knew very well that the regulatory environment within which my business could grow did not allow enough space for my vision. Like thousands of hair renegades like myself, I have not let the threat of legal sanction stop me from acting on my calling. If you are like me, I encourage you to do the same!

Chapter 7
"So, HOW DID YOU COME UP WITH THIS IDEA ANYWAY?"

Those who know me as an academic are usually surprised to learn that I also do hair. In fact, some would say I lead a double life. The academic by day, I'm lecturing, teaching, meeting and talking with colleagues and community folks. It's a full and gratifying existence all of its own, to be sure! By night, off come the suit and pumps, and on go the Tee-shirt and tennies, and the Sisterlocks lady is behind someone's chair, locking and sharing real-people talk, or in front of a computer trying to figure out how to make a business out of a lofty vision. Or, I'm working up a demonstration for a beauty college or talking to someone long distance about how to keep those locks from unraveling at the ends.

I've always been a believer in developing transferable skills, and I can truly say that I practice what I preach. What I have lived and learned as the Sisterlocks lady has served me very well in keeping an activist edge on my academic work, which in turn has helped me tremendously in developing Sisterlocks, both as a philosophy and as a business.

In any case, **no matter what role I might be carrying out at any given moment, the same hair follows me day and night,** and speaks volumes about who I really am! When I stand before a university committee, I am still a sister from Detroit with tight, African-textured locks. When I walk into a community function where alas, my sisters are still seriously grappling with chemical dependency, my hair is a loving, if not so subtle call for us all to look deeply into our reflections in the mirror each day for our true image. My profession does not alter who I am, and I do not alter what I look like. In all of this, I have always found the simple fact that our hair will always bring us back to our 'bottom line,' extremely intriguing. It has been both a blessing and a curse for our women as we have tried in many different ways to make our mark in this country.

When people learn that I teach about Africa they often ask if the Sisterlocks concept came to me as a result of knowledge I picked up about hair practices. It would be great if I could claim to have re-activated a lost African adornment tradition, but this was not the case. In fact, in most of the African cultures I know about, hair locking techniques are not generally practiced. When people wear locks, they tend to be associated with specific religious cults.

Though women traditionally wear a host of short and medium natural styles, these are usually twisted, wrapped, plaited or sculpted into artistic shapes. For longer styles, before the advent of the foreign hair extension industry, added extensions made of natural fibers were used.

Although I can not claim to have been called by an African deity to carry out this good work for our women, I can assert that there is something deeply spiritual about what I do. The type of spirituality I experience

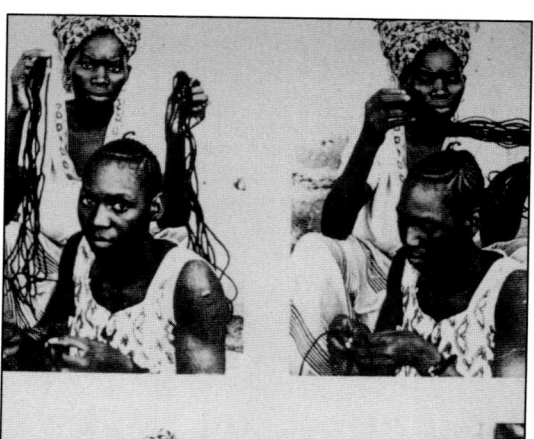

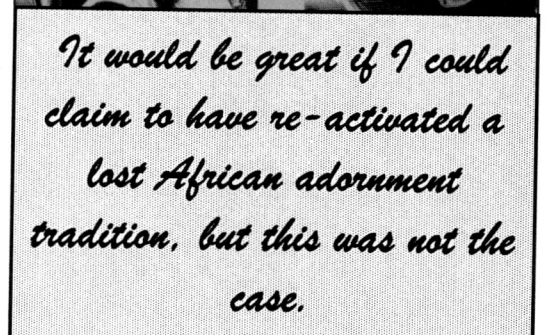

> *It would be great if I could claim to have re-activated a lost African adornment tradition, but this was not the case.*

through sharing Sisterlocks with others is not connected to any specific belief system or religion, though. Nonetheless, it often pervades my interactions with clients in an almost tangible way. Most often, these are people - both male and female - who are in the process of embracing their sense of self in a way that they never have done before. They are beginning to look deep inside for answers to long-held, unanswered questions. They are becoming courageous enough to love themselves, sometimes after a lifetime of feeling under-valued. They are becoming strong enough to be self-critical, and learning how to live in a manner more true to their nature.

I often say Sisterlocks is not about a hairdo. It is about a way of life, and a process of re-defining oneself on a very deep and spiritual level. There is tremendous power in that redefinition. Those who take that step are ready to take on the last frontier of self-love and self-acceptance. They are soul searching and finding ways to heal themselves. This is a movement that is gaining momentum, and will soon be unstoppable!

There was no way, ten or fifteen years ago, that I could have imagined myself ever owning a natural hair care business that would play a vital role in ending what I call the 'aesthetic crisis' our women have been steeped in for several generations. As I reflect on the aspects of my life that finally synthesized around the Sisterlocks idea, I realize that there were several factors at work.

For example, I have always been obsessed with my hair. Now, I realize that it is not unusual for young girls to become more conscious of their appearance as they gain a keener awareness of the people and attitudes around them, but I think you will grant me that four years old is

> *I often say Sisterlocks is not about a hairdo. It is about a way of life, and a process of re-defining oneself on a very deep and spiritual level. There is tremendous power in that redefinition.*

a little early to launch a hair styling career. I mean, nobody could do my hair right but me. By that age, I could already braid (or so I thought), and the only thing I lacked was the authority to dismiss the adults around me who insisted on messing with my creations. The biggest offenders were my mother and grandmother, salon owners and beauticians, who of course thought they knew what they were doing!

I grew up in beauty salons, and quite frankly, I disliked them intensely!

I almost never got what I wanted in a hairdo there, and I almost never saw anything I would have wanted on the other ladies' heads as they left the salons either. However, in these places where necessary evils were carried out, I did learn many of the important skills of the trade. I can remember my grandmother teaching me the 'right way' to wield a curling iron, for example, and how to finger-wave. I was still a pre-teen at the time. I learned the fine points of hot combing too, but this was done by trial and error on myself, my sisters and mom at home. (ouch!) By the time I was a young adult, I had taught myself every new chemical technique out. I became the resident beautician wherever I went. When I went off to college, I took my trade with me. My late night beauty parlor activities have saved many a black coed from embarrassment in those days when you would die before letting them know that you had to straighten your hair to get it like theirs. Sisters came to me when the humidity had gotten to their 'dos, when their roots were causing their hair to break off or when they simply wanted me to snatch up that kitchen. Oh, I could tame me some Mother Nature!

By the time I was in my late 20s, like many African American women, I was sick to death of relying on all of the magic tricks that seemed to be required of me in order to make myself acceptable to both others and myself. I knew that locks were an alternative, but I had never seen any done in a way that suited me. Most of the women I saw looked as if their locks were wearing THEM rather than the other way around. I never seriously considered locks for myself until I began seeing professional women at conferences year after year. Each time I saw them, their locks would look more and more stunning. This was the period I call my "wanna-be" stage. I loved the way the locks looked on these other women, but I as yet lacked the courage to try locks on my own hair. Mind you I had worn a short natural for many years, but like most women, I could only relate to my natural hair when it was short and 'manageable.' During this entire period, braids were becoming more and more popular, and more commonly seen on women from all walks of life. I am sure that this, combined with my admiration of locks on other women, gave me the courage to decide to try locks for myself.

The decision was made! But it took me two more years to get up the courage to try them! Even then, I chose to start growing my natural locks under the cover of extensions. About every 2 months I would undo and re-tighten the extensions, and in the process, monitor the growth of what I believed to be my pre-locked natural hair. When I had let my hair grow for about 8 months, I started gradually eliminating the extensions, which I'd had made very small. At that point I began experimenting with ways of keeping my natural locks very small and avoiding the common problems of bunching and breakage.

Believe me, I met with a lot of set backs here. The main problem was that I discovered my hair had not really locked while in braids (twists, actually). Yes, it had matted in spots, but the tight structure of the extension hair had kept my own hair's natural interlocking process from taking over.

On the positive side, going through this process of growing my natural hair under the cover of extensions was making me feel very much at home with it. I worked diligently over the next year or so to come up with a way to make my full, very expressive mid-length natural hair with relaxed ends, more stylable.

Finally, I had taken all of the extensions out and I (kind of) had the look I wanted. The next problem I faced was that each time I went into the shower

> *During this entire period, braids were becoming more and more popular, and more commonly seen on women from all walks of life.*

to wash my hair it just bunched up like mad! I would end up spending hours stretching and twisting my locks back out. I had to keep them wet during this process, because if they dried out in that state I never would have been able to pull or rip the lumps out. At one point I resorted to washing my hair on rollers to keep the locks smooth and controlled during the washing process. I would roll my hair up, shampoo it, unroll each roller and thoroughly towel dry the section, then re-roll it. After three hours (!!@#%!!) I was ready to sit under a dryer for another hour - minimum. Needless to say I had to find a better way, or just cut the s--- off.

I was going through a lot of intense feelings about my hair during that phase. On my good days I was determined to see this experiment through and not give up on my natural hair. On my bad days I was constantly fighting back the urge to give into that old lie about our hair being not exactly real hair at all, but rather some kind of curse that made us not quite as good as everybody else.

> *I kept at it. I realized that my natural hair type was clearly not designed to be combed.*

I knew I had to detach myself from my feelings about my hair in order to be able to analyze and solve the issues logically. I tried imagining myself to be a Martian with no emotional attachment whatsoever to the meanings my hair held for me - meanings that made me so self conscious I couldn't even think. Maybe the solutions would come then.

This detachment thing was very hard for me though, because my hair for me was not just some malleable neutral material that could be made to conform to my will. It spoke to me of my past, my family, my culture, and all of the things I had never resolved in my life. Thank goodness I'm so stubborn! I kept at it. I realized that my natural hair type was clearly not designed to be combed. Any coily-structured material will respond better to hand-shaping, twisting and weaving procedures than it will to those that seek to flatten it out. I finally settled on the weaving idea, but I just couldn't come up with anything that topped the braid. I knew I still wasn't thinking about the problem in quite the right way.

I can remember the day I successfully locked on to the necessary mind set. (Pun intended.) I was watching someone's hands. They were gesturing about how to weave the strands of a rope and I remembered that multi-strand weaving is not always done from the base to the tip, but also in some cases from the tip to the base. I must have latched on to a memory of some of the weaving gadgets we played with as kids. Not just knitting and crocheting, but all manner of thimble and loom shaped contraptions seem to have fallen into our hands. With these toys I looped yarn into many an article that defied description, but that my mother always loved.

Working with these toys successfully instilled in me a tactile understanding of many weaving principles. Connecting with this understanding provided the final key to the problem I was grappling with; how to create tiny braid-like structures in hair that, unlike braids, would not have to be taken out as the hair grew. Working from the tip to the roots would accomplish this.

I had my concept down, and I was ready to try it on myself. Now, I have to describe to you the condition of my hair at this time. I had relaxed ends that melded into quite lumpy but still relatively small locked sections of hair that, as you got closer to the root area, exploded into loose, natural tufts of hair. I'm telling you, I was going on faith! I carefully 'locked' this loose area in each section of hair by passing the tip of the hair through this loose part, moving in several directions. Compared to today's Sisterlocks standards, my technique was really crude, but when I'd finished, that section of each lock looked more uniform than the rest. However, I knew that the real test would come when I washed my hair.

I went a couple of days before that fateful shampooing. I knew I would be risking having to start from scratch again, and I wanted to enjoy my hair a little first! I was more than a bit nervous when I finally stepped into the shower to shampoo my hair. I'm sure I washed it very gently, but honestly, I don't remember anything about the experience. What I do remember is getting out of the shower and going straight to the mirror to check on whether my new technique had survived it's maiden voyage. **I couldn't believe it.** My locks looked exactly the way they had looked when I'd gotten into the shower. No more lumpy than before, and they hadn't shrunk up or blown out. They were just sitting there.... I don't know how much time passed before I could react to what I was seeing.

It couldn't be this simple.

It was almost embarrassing. What I had done all of a sudden seemed so obvious, so logical that I couldn't believe it had not been thought of before.

I remained in this incredulous state for quite some time - days, I think. I kept inspecting my locks for signs that their integrity was degrading, but ... nothing! They just stayed neat! My state of near-disbelief gradually turned into elation. I was almost afraid to give over to what I was truly feeling. It seemed too big for me. Those around me began to notice my hair more. I began to experience what women today who get Sisterlocks routinely experience. I couldn't be out in public without being stopped with questions, compliments, strange people staring at, or actually wanting to touch my hair. They all had the same questions: *"Are they just little braids?" "How do you do that?" "Can you take them out?" "Is that really your hair?"* and on and on. Many women with braids tell me they get these reactions too, but the fact that this was my Natural hair was a difficult concept for most women to process. I began to 'complain,' but I loved the attention my hair was getting. It was the kind of confirmation I needed for my belief that I was really on to something with this technique.

More than any other reactions, those of African American women really gripped me. To borrow a phrase from Zora Neale Hurston, it was like something fell off the shelf inside them when they saw my hair. I knew that look. I understood it deeply. I had felt what they were feeling a million times. It is a combination of fear and longing that is so strong it will instantly set you off your center.

I got so that I could pretty well judge a Black woman's mind set by the length of time she stared at my hair. Some women recovered quickly from the force of their feelings, especially if they weren't ready to face what the spectacle of my hair brought up inside them. These women tended to look for something to negate the power of what they felt by asking things like "What if you want to go back to your own hair?" I took this to mean relaxed. I've even had women unconsciously refer to their hair in its relaxed state as "normal."

Most black women wouldn't say anything at all, but simply couldn't take their eyes off my hair. I could feel their stares if they were sitting out of my gaze; If they could be seen, they would try to sneak peeks as best they could; If we were talking face to face, they would really be talking to my hair, not focusing on my person. These were usually the women who had gone at least part way down the road to accepting their own natural hair. They were like the "wanna-be" I used to be. Then there were the women who were comfortable commenting on, or

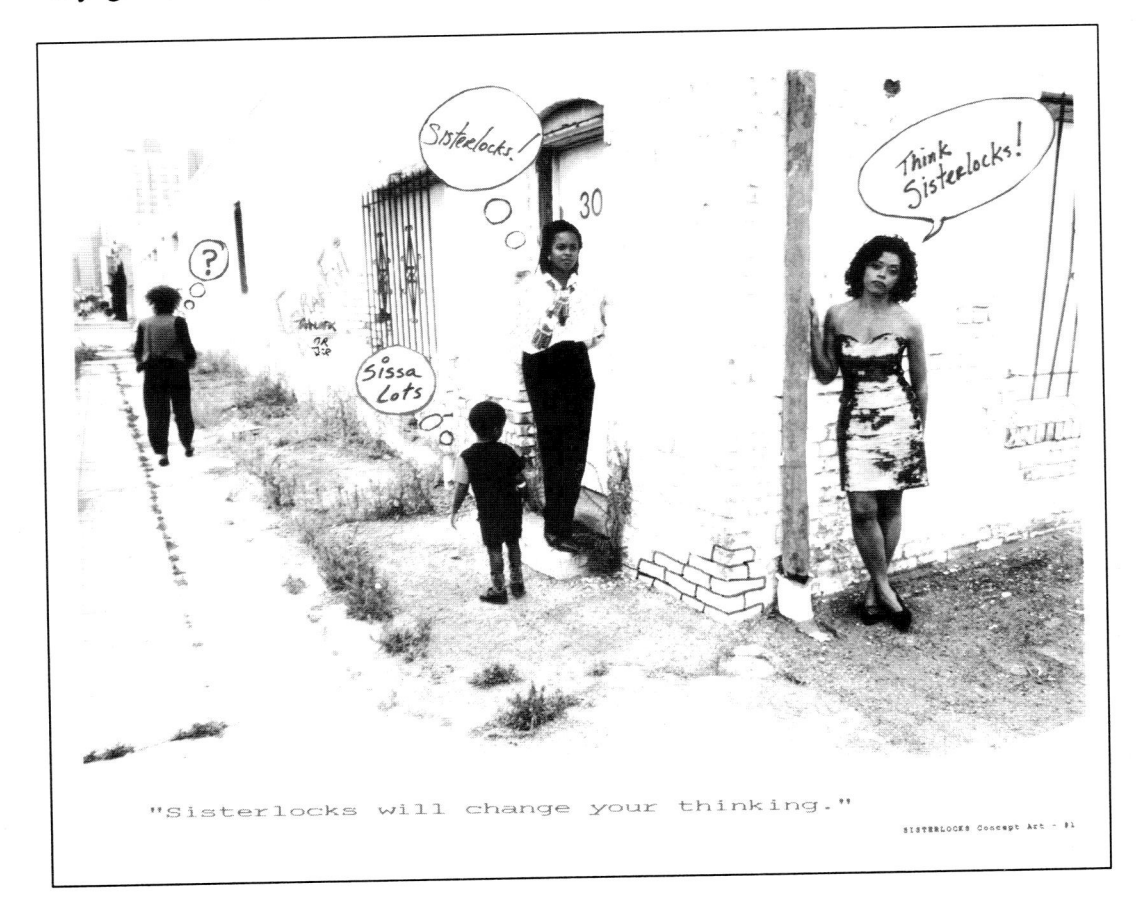

"Sisterlocks will change your thinking."

complementing my look. These were the women who either had worn, were wearing, or would soon wear a natural look themselves.

The men were looking too, and talking! Overall, they were less inhibited than the women, and would actually volunteer compliments about my hair - something I'd never experienced before. Virtually all of the reactions I got confirmed how much power this 'hair thing' holds for us as a people. This was especially true for our women who, practically without exception, reacted to my hair on a deep level. All of the anxieties I had ever felt about myself and my hair were echoed in the faces of the women I encountered over that first year of Sisterlocks. That is how I came to the

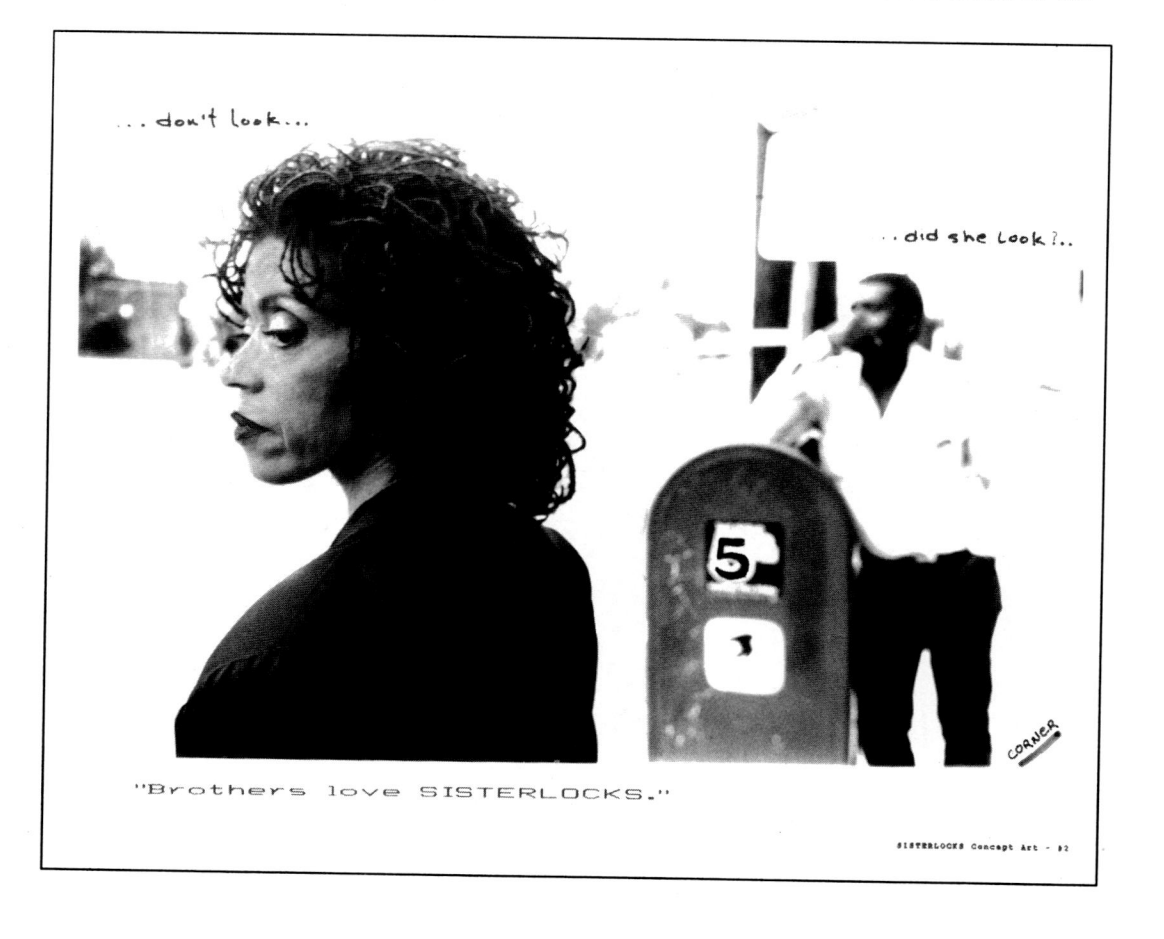

"Brothers love SISTERLOCKS."

feeling that I had been given a calling.

Receiving a calling is a strange and wonderful thing. I'm not sure exactly how to talk about it, because it is not something that happens the same way to everyone. For me, it has been like being in a state of abandon, but without the recklessness you would normally expect. I feel very calm, but at the same time I feel absolutely fearless in taking on whatever challenges come my way. There is no place in my mind for the thought that the Sisterlocks vision will not be realized. Nothing I can imagine feels too great to face, and I know with absolute certainty that the outcome will be positive. What a high!

Obviously, with this new perspective, my sense of purpose changed. Though I loved the uniqueness of my hair, I realized that this was not just something for me alone. In the beginning I would play-complain to my companion, who was often with me in public to witness the reactions my hair received from other women. "I should carry brochures!," I would lament to him after having to answer the same questions over and over again. I went from saying this jokingly to taking it seriously, and without knowing much at all about business, I knew I had to start one.

Mind you, these feelings came to me before I had done anyone else's hair at all! Fortunately, not too long thereafter my sister, Carol, announced she wanted her hair like mine. Unfortunately for Carol though, I didn't have the slightest idea what I was doing. I had assumed that I could simply do what I had done on my own hair, but since she had a different texture, nothing was coming out like I had planned. It was on my sister's hair that I learned the importance of things like choosing the right locking sizes; parting appropriately; varying the locking pattern to the specific texture and density of the hair. When I think about it today, I can't believe she trusted me with her magnificent head of hair! She had an extremely well cared for relaxer that was shoulder length. She had a beautician she loved and who kept her hair healthy and well manicured. What gave her the courage to become my guinea pig, I will never understand! I'm sure that my 'learning curve' cost her about a year of hair growth, but she hung in there with me.

Because of Carol and my 5 or 6 next 'victims', the Sisterlocks approach evolved from a technique to a full-blown hair care system. I

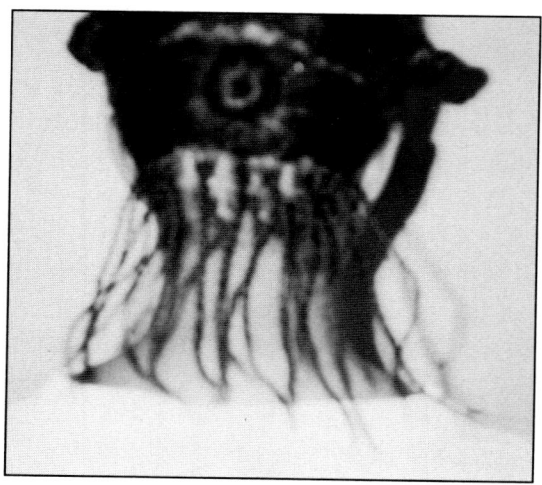

I learned a lot from mistakes I made - like making parting sizes too large. Too much scalp shows, and locks can bunch!

couldn't believe it, but each new head I did was different in some way, and none of them was like mine. I felt like screaming, "Could I please just get a sister with a head full of tight, kinky hair!" But, no-o-o! I got hair that was extremely smooth, hair that was extremely soft and thin, hair with an extremely deep coil to it, hair that was excessively stiff, you name it! Each time, I had to adjust my approach to meet the challenges posed by that particular hair type.

I gave away a lot of free time in those days, re-doing locks, undoing bunching and matting, splitting or combining locks, working with those hairlines, but I was learning the whole time. One thing I learned was that an understanding of the full range of our hair types was a necessary prerequisite for doing Sisterlocks, and this became part of the standard approach to teaching the system to others. I also developed techniques for dealing with the specific problems I had to work through.

For example, I soon realized that I needed tools for locking the hair neatly to the scalp. I first tried a crocheting hook, which was the right concept, but the wrong shape. Not only does it tug unnecessarily at the scalp, it is cumbersome and slows the operator down. I've heard that some enterprising sister has even come up with a weed-wacker-looking implement that yanks the hair through the open spaces to create the locks! Not good for creating uniform locks! Also not good for the tender-headed, or those with fragile hair types! If somebody comes at you with one of these instruments of torture, beware! They probably don't have the skill level or the proper training needed to give you a professional job with good long-term results! The tools I designed reflect what I learned from years of problem solving, They take into consideration both locking efficiency and customer comfort.

After working through these kinds of problems, I thought I was ready for the big leagues, and from a technical standpoint, I was. But I was not ready for the attitudes and questionable practices I discovered to be the norm once I stepped out into the professional arena. I went gaily tripping into East and West Coast salons, both traditional ones and those for natural hair care. I wanted to showcase my system and learn what the professional reactions might be. At the time I was literally ready to lay this in the lap of someone within the industry who could take it to the next level. Well, I discovered that nobody wanted it! The traditional salons generally saw it as a threat to their business. I was actually told this to my face in a San Francisco establishment. The natural hair salons were more generous in their acceptance of the idea, except for a few lock extremists who continue to view Sisterlocks as imitation, "instant locks," as one beautifully locked, but vehement sister put it.

Overall though, the established natural salons didn't seem the least bit interested at first in making Sisterlocks a part of their trade. This confused me a lot before I understood the economics of salon management as it is taught from the cosmetologist's perspective. Simply stated, salons have difficulty making a profit on lengthy procedures. This goes for the natural salons as

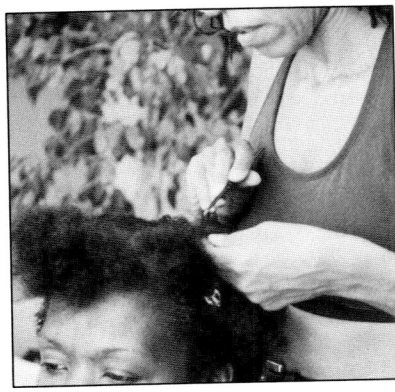

An early crochet hook victim

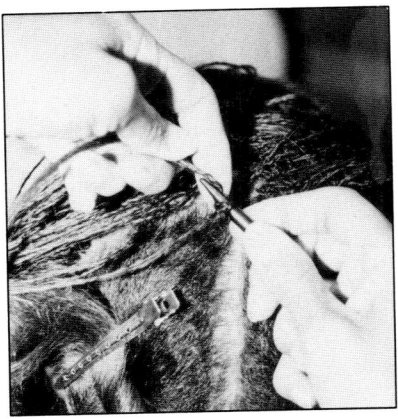

One of the Sisterlocks tools

> *I also learned that some people who claim to want to bring professionalism -ism to the natural hair care industry resent having to go through the kind of serious training that Sisterlocks involves.*

well. They may be 'down' with the sisters, but when it is all said and done, they use basically the same customer service criteria to meet their overhead as traditional salons. This means that they have to select their services based on whether or not these will generate a pre-determined profit margin.

My little adventure taught me that I would simply have to do everything myself: Establish a training program; Create a demand for Sisterlocks by getting it 'out there' and seen; Educate the public about what to expect from the system and from the practitioner claiming to do Sisterlocks; Establish some legal protection against those who would try to steal or misrepresent the idea, or downgrade the quality of the system.

This last point has really been important because I've discovered that not everyone in the industry puts quality first and does business with integrity. For example, I have had established salons give out all kinds of misinformation about what Sisterlocks are and what they will do, instead of referring questions to the company, or finding out for themselves about the system. I want the readers of this work to know that Sisterlocks does not do business in this way. When someone calls the home office with questions about braided extensions, they are referred to braiding professionals who are known to have a good reputation. If someone wants cosmetology services - hair coloring for example - they are referred to a reputable salon.

I also learned that some people who claim to want to bring professionalism to the natural hair care industry resent having to go through the kind of serious training that Sisterlocks involves. They want to look over someone's shoulder and "get it" in 10 minutes, so that

THEY can go out and start making money for themselves. Don't they know that our women deserve more than to be subjected to practitioners with just a superficial knowledge of any system?

There are also scores of people - among them, the very women for whom the Sisterlocks gift is intended - who are just waiting to steal (Can you believe it?!) the Sisterlocks system, despite the fact that it is trademarked, and offer a BRAND X version that they think will bring them more money. "You can't trademark a hair system" they spit. They don't see that the trademark approach is for the protection of the CUSTOMER! It is not meant as a challenge to others within the industry. It is meant to help professionalize it.

I have had people with an ounce of training try to hang up their shingle as Certified Sisterlocks professionals. I have had people with 2 ounces of training go out and set up copy-cat training programs of their own. What discourages me is that our women have come to expect so little in the way of quality hair care, that pseudo-professionals can get away with this kind of deceit. Unfortunately for those who fall for their scams, they usually get inferior quality and empty promises, but rarely lower prices.

Have these experiences discouraged me? Not in the least. As I move through the world, I am daily reminded of the power of this vision that is unfolding. The experiences I relate here have made me all the more determined to stand behind my structured, professional approach that puts the needs of our women first. **Our women deserve the assurance of high standards and an approach that is a celebration of our sisterhood.** This will always be the driving force behind the Sisterlocks idea. Count on it!

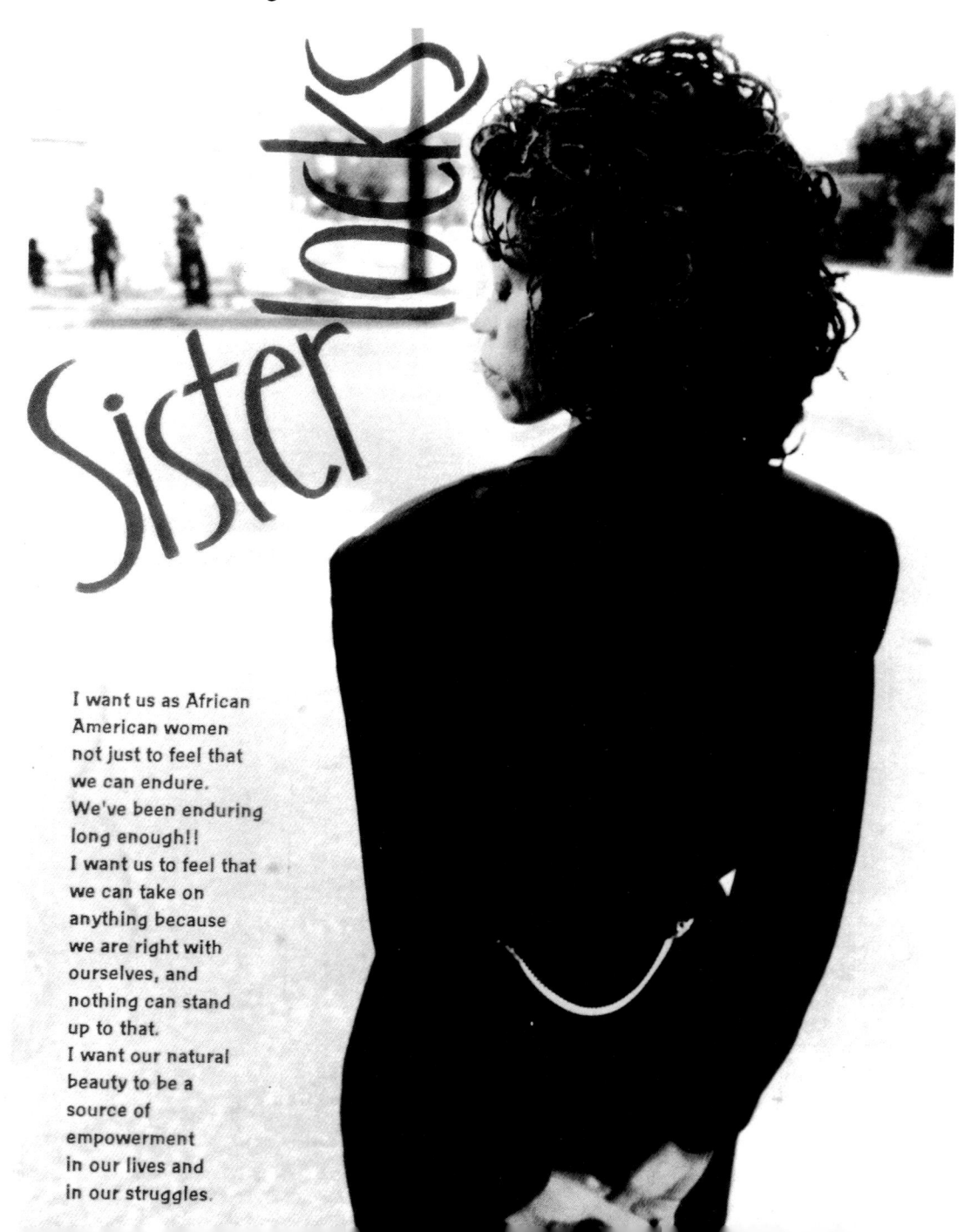

Sisterlocks

I want us as African American women not just to feel that we can endure. We've been enduring long enough!! I want us to feel that we can take on anything because we are right with ourselves, and nothing can stand up to that. I want our natural beauty to be a source of empowerment in our lives and in our struggles.

Chapter 8
THE SISTERLOCKS APPROACH

As a child sitting at my mother's feet to get my hair combed and plaited, I was not aware of the tradition that was being carried forward in our home. West African hair artistry was not even something I could pronounce back then, let alone contemplate. My world was a few square blocks in a Black working class Detroit neighborhood. By my time in mid 20th century America, the meaning and holistic nature of African women's traditional hair care had become all but lost to my people. Certain gestures still remained, but for most of us these had lost their deep meaning. The experience of feeling connected through hair styling to more important things like our history and cultural values, had certainly been lost. All I knew was that the kinks hurt when my mother combed them, and I never much liked the styles that came out of what felt to me like a ritual form of torture!

Its ironic how today, I relish the hours I spend with the women (and men) whose hair I work on. Its a real bonding time. We laugh and joke, catch up on each other's business, discuss life and love, listen to music. Sometimes my customers are put to sleep by the massaging sensation of having their hair locked or re-tightened. I massage their shoulders when they've been sitting too long; They kick off their shoes and make themselves more

> *As a child sitting at my mother's feet to get my hair combed and plaited, I was not aware of the tradition that was being carried forward in our home.*

"to home;" We visit with people passing through. By the end of their hours with me, they go away with more than a hairdo. We have shared a piece of our lives in that time, and our shared experience has become part of what their hairdo signifies in their lives.

Dealing with the whole person is at the heart of the Sisterlocks approach, and this is the main reason why I insist the people I train use a consultation to get to know both the people and the hair they will be working on. Doing the hair is not treated as just an isolated event - just some kind of transaction where money is exchanged for a service. The customer is honored as a person with both a past and a future, and the Sisterlocks experience entwines itself with both. The hair issues that bring the client to the Sisterlocks Consultant's chair in the first place, are probably the same ones the consultant has dealt with at some time too. Understanding a client's personal hair history gives insight into why the person wants locks in the first place, and what they expect the locks to do for them. The consultant needs to understand these things, because they will determine how the locks are to be done: Larger for those with hurried lifestyles, or for those who can't be bothered primping and pruning their hair; Smaller for the very style-conscious; More time for that sister who is impatient by nature, and will need more supervision getting through the settling-in phase; More explanation for that brother who had a bad experience with traditional locks, and so is going to need a clearer understanding of the hair's natural interlocking process.

The client's future is also at stake when they get Sisterlocks. Their hair becomes a more prominent feature of their appearance, and a greater factor in how they are seen by others, as well as their self-perception. The consultant and client enter into a relationship of trust based on the assurance that the consultant will keep the locks looking beautiful over time, adjust the look as needed, correct problems that arise, and teach the client what to do to gain more of a sense of control over their looks. This is why I stress that clients choose their consultants well! Sometimes in their impatience to get the Sisterlocks, they feel they must put up with someone who is not fully competent in the system, or simply whose personality is not compatible with their own. If Sisterlocks is new in their area, they may not have a choice in the beginning.

Just remember, the consultant/client relationship is the biggest single factor in the long-term success of the Sisterlocks. Don't entrust your hair to a hack! Fully certified consultants maintain an ongoing relationship with the home office, and have access to technical advise, problem solving tips and re-training opportunities. When we get ongoing complaints about a particular consultant, we drop them from our referral registry. This means that a client can phone us at any time to find out if their consultant is in good standing, or to praise or express concern about any problem.

I admit, I have been accused of being a maniac about the quality control aspect of this hair care system. "You can't control what other people do," is the line I've heard a million times. Just because I'd like to personally oversee every Sisterlocks job in the entire country, to ensure that everyone's hair ends up looking as gorgeous as mine... Just because I want to hand-train every professional and have them apprentice with **me** until their skills are perfect... Just because I'd like to control everyone's pricing, and direct their marketing campaigns,... (is that being a maniac???) Seriously though, what I see daily is that our women have been taken advantage of so much and for so long that many of us have actually given up hope. We don't think we can have it all - luxurious hair that is OUR OWN, and fair prices from competent, well trained professionals.

True, I can't control what other people do, but I believe that providing people with the best information about what is possible will result in raised expectations. In my experience as an educator, raised expectations

> *Just remember, the consultant - client relationship is the biggest single factor in the long-term success of the Sisterlocks Don't entrust your hair to a hack!*

result in higher performance levels. You will get more only if you do not settle for less! So, I want to devote the remainder of this chapter to an illustration of what the Sisterlocks experience can be like, and along the way, answer a few of the general questions asked by people wanting to know more about Sisterlocks, or wanting to learn the system. What kind of women want Sisterlocks? What is the process like? What is it like to have Sisterlocks? What long-term results can someone expect?

What kinds of people get Sisterlocks?

Most of my customers are women, though I also have several Brotherlocks clients. I can say that ALL kinds of women get them, but there is a certain general type that will get them **first**. These are the sisters with enough self confidence to step out ahead of others, and by their actions, they influence the decisions of their peers. Most of the women in this core group are independent minded and self-loving and interested in self-empowerment. Oh yes, and they are usually pretty sassy! When they get Sisterlocks though, they get even sassier! Even the soft spoken ones get 'that attitude.' This comes from the experience of finally finding something that helps them celebrate who they really are. In most cases, these women have been looking for a way to wear their hair that is consistent with their need to feel genuine about themselves. They have felt dissatisfied and frustrated at having to rely on the limited range of hair care systems for our women, all of which they felt were demeaning in some way.

I would certainly put Maria in this category. I'll be using her pictures to illustrate this section. Though fairly soft spoken, she is an intense young woman who had been uncomfortable with her hair care options for quite a long time. When she heard about Sisterlocks, she headed with all deliberate speed to one of our training sessions where she modeled for a demo-consultation. When we teach the Sisterlocks system, we make sure that our trainees learn more than just the technique. We teach them how to prepare prospective clients, how to deliver the services effectively with customer comfort in mind, and how to maintain healthy locks over time.

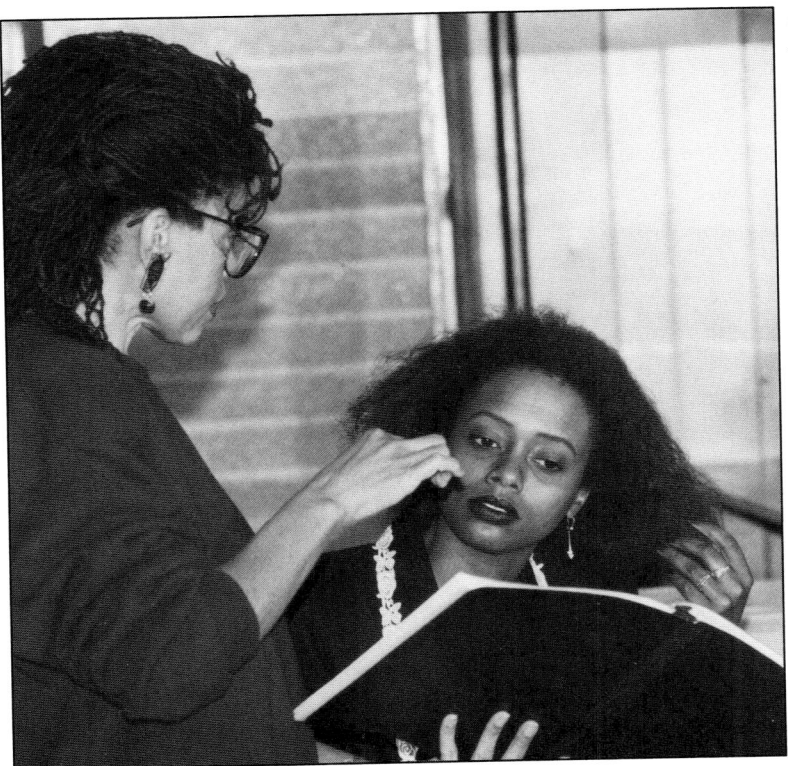

What is the process like?

The standard Sisterlocks system is offered as a package of three visits: the consultation; the locking session; the follow-up visit. At times I have gotten clients who become impatient with the idea of a consultation. They think they know what they want, and they just want to pay their money to get it. I believe that some of them even suspect that a consultation is just a way to get extra money from customers. With the Sisterlocks system though, we make the consultation mandatory, so ladies, don't blame your Consultants. They're just doing their jobs. In truth though, no responsible professional would apply a system to someone's hair that is virtually permanent, without doing a consultation first.

The trained Sisterlocks Consultant uses the consultation to learn about the hair care history of the client, examine the type and condition of the client's hair, and fully inform the client about what to expect from the Sisterlocks system. After that, the consultant puts a few sample locks in the client's hair, testing different sizes and types of locks. The client will live in the locks for a couple of weeks, making sure to shampoo them once or twice to determine how they will behave and exactly which way of doing the locks is best. This process gives the consultant the necessary information to do the best job possible, and also educates the client and involves them in the decision making process.

A consultation is not a guarantee of satisfaction, but it comes closer than anything else I know of.

Believe me, both the consultant and the client want to do everything they can to avoid the client breaking down in tears after the all-day locking session has just been completed. (Yes, this really happened!) I can testify that the vast majority of women whose hair I have locked go through an anxiety attack of some sort. The reasons for this relate to all of the issues I go into in the first part of this book. Usually, the attack occurs shortly before they come in to be locked - sometimes the day before, sometimes a few hours before. If they make it in for their appointment, they're usually over the hump.

An accomplished consultant can complete a head of average-length hair (4-5 inches) in 8 to 10 hours, but when first learning the techniques, it can easily take a consultant several hours longer. These new consultants are usually quite good, and the more heads they do, the faster they get. If the client needs frequent breaks, the job can also take longer. If the consultant is working with an assistant it will take a shorter amount of time. In my experience, working more than two on a head decreases both efficiency and quality.

The Sisterlocks system gives the consultant guidelines for every phase of the locking process including sectioning the hair, establishing the appropriate parting sizes for the locks, establishing the proper tension within each lock, and deciding when to use which locking tools. Customer comfort is always stressed.

Getting Sisterlocks should not be torture for the client! If the consultant has an adequate level of skill, a mild tug from time to time is all the client will feel. I invite my own customers to let me know if I get too rough, then I adjust my touch accordingly. Strange, but I find that if I don't extend the invitation to speak up, most women will not volunteer feed back about their level of comfort. Many of us just assume we have to put up with pain when getting our hair done. Not so with Sisterlocks. Our system does not require that the hair be tightly secured at the scalp, as with many techniques that add extensions or wefts of hair.

When the locks are first put in, they are thinner and stiffer than

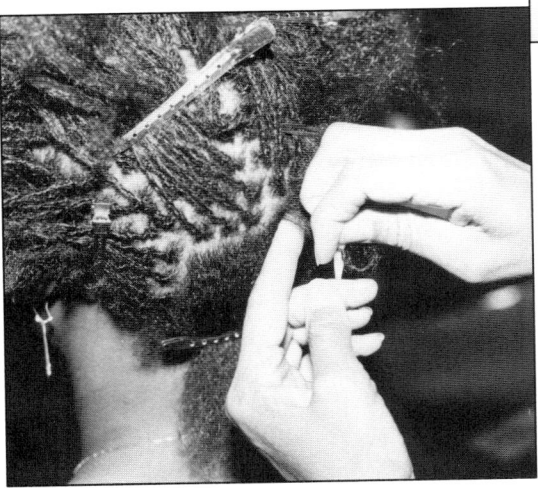

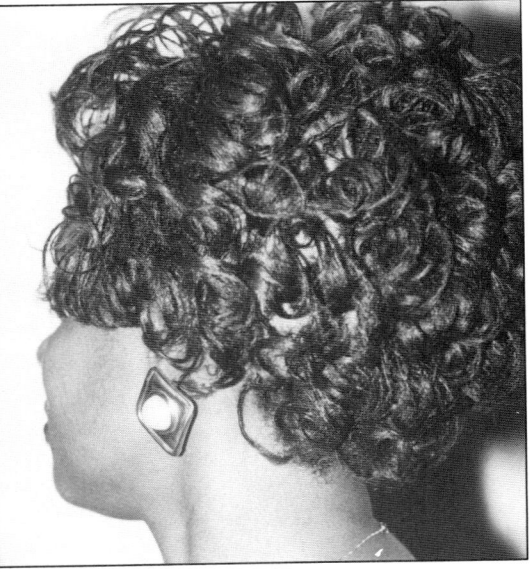

Freshly locked and styled

The locking process (relaxed ends left loose)

normal, and look like tiny braids. Depending on the thickness of the hair, there will be some scalp showing. The locks thicken and fill in with a couple of shampooings though, as the hair's natural texture begins to express itself. I tell my customers who are feeling a little insecure at this stage that if they LIKE their hair even a little bit at this stage, they will absolutely LOVE it as their locks thicken and mature. I am still waiting to be proven wrong on this point.

The settling-in phase is next. This is the period during which the hair shifts around in response to washing and styling, and decides where **it** wants to settle within the locking structure of Sisterlocks. During the consultation, clients learn how to properly shampoo

> No heavy, oil-based products on the locks, ever!

their hair, and what to watch for as the locks settle. The duration of the settling phase varies greatly depending on the length, texture and condition of the hair. It can be as short as 3 weeks, or as long as 6 months, or even longer in extreme cases. With time, consultants get pretty good at accurately predicting how long the client will have to follow the special care procedures when washing, grooming and styling. It is possible for the locks to bunch or unravel during this phase. This usually happens when clients get too care free with their Sisterlocks too soon, or when consultants are too lenient with guidelines or not specific enough in their instructions. Problems that arise during the settling phase can almost always be corrected, if caught in time.

I find that one of the toughest instructions for our folks to follow is the one that says "No heavy, oil-based products on the locks, ever!" This is especially important during the settling-in phase when this can cause the locks to slip excessively. The locks are meant to be permanent, and so nothing should be applied that will not easily wash out with each shampooing. Many of us desperately want our hair to shine as though it were naturally straight hair, and have always relied on grease to try to achieve this. The Sisterlocks approach has a completely different focus. It says that clean, healthy natural hair will have its own natural luster. For some hair types, this luster will be deeper than others. Once the locks have settled, we recommend only light oil-based

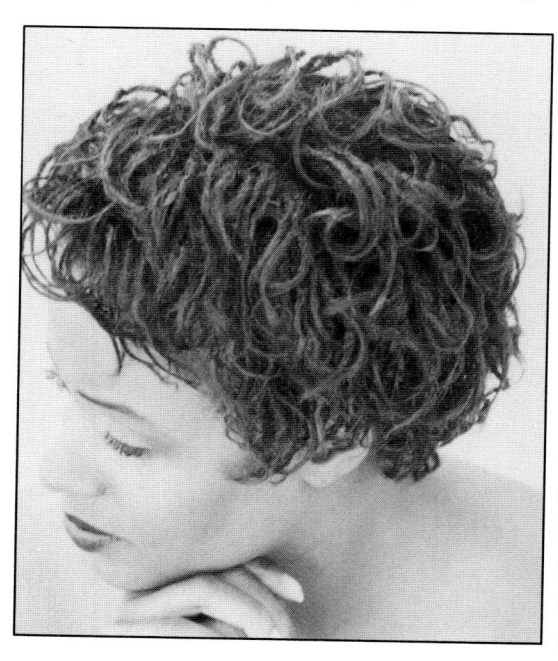

Locks settled in - filled in

products, or non-oily products containing humectants that are non-sticky and non-residue producing. Locks that are oily or impacted do not hold a set well, and can even develop hard spots that result in weakened locks over time.

Our own product line is of course ideal for the Sisterlocks, and for any 'leave-in' style, including braid extensions and weaves applied to the natural hair. I discovered very early that most products marketed to African American women are formulated to fit the needs of processed hair. Some leave a coating on the hair either to give the temporary appearance of a shine, or to de-tangle the hair. With the locks, we WANT the hair's natural coiliness to fully express itself, so de-tangling is not desired.

Our products focus on deep-cleaning and conditioning the hair so it stays healthy and produces its own natural luster. Products formulated for processed hair must correct for the partial damage to the hair shafts already caused by the chemicals themselves. They must try not to further aggravate this with the cleaning agents they use. (They are not always successful, by the way.) Mature, well cared-for Sisterlocks are light and very responsive to styling. Cut into one, and you will find nothing collecting inside! It's the cleanest, most versatile locking system yet devised.

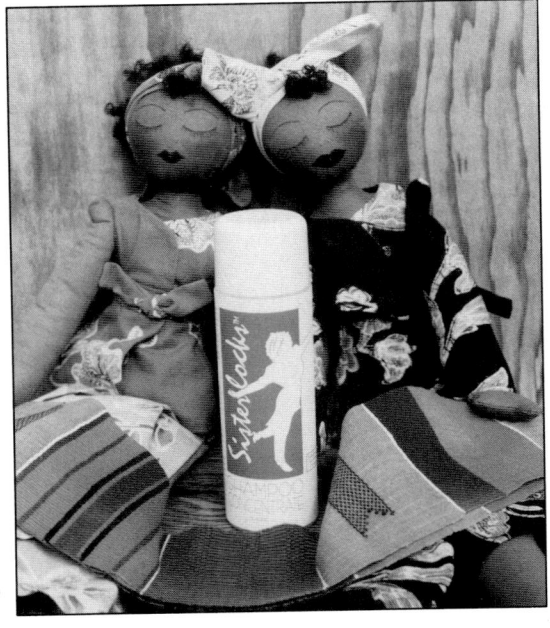

Sisterlocks custom products - ideal for locks, braids and all naturally-textured hair.

At some time during the settling phase, the client will see the consultant for a follow-up visit. Like the consultation, this is a mandatory part of the Sisterlocks package. This is a time for tightening everything up, correcting slippage, troubleshooting if necessary, and re-advising the client about procedures. By this time the client should be able to maintain her hair properly between re-tightening sessions. After my clients have had their locks for 6 months or so, they are eligible to take my re-tightening class so they can have more control over maintaining their locks between visits. I advise them to still see me 2 or 3 times a year however, to check things out and get a professional grooming. This system works very well, as Maria will tell you.

What is it like to have Sisterlocks?

Women report that having Sisterlocks brings a lot of attention their way. This attention is overwhelmingly positive, and much of it comes from men. The Brotherlocks fellows experience similar reactions from both men and women. If you're considering Sisterlocks, expect to be the talk of your workplace, class, church group or whatever. Expect unsolicited compliments from men and women of every possible description. It may surprise you to learn that many of my customers report that they receive more positive comments from Caucasians in their environments than they do from African Americans. Interesting, huh? They also report that the people who are stand-offish in the beginning usually warm up as the locks grow longer, fuller and more impressive. (You know, that long hair thing!)

Women (and men) begin a love affair with their natural hair that is healing and empowering. They feel the impact of an improved relationship with their hair in every aspect of their lives. They talk about hair more. They notice other peoples' hair more. And, oh by the way, almost without exception, they all succumb to the **Sisterlocks Disease!!!** This is the inability to keep their hands out of their hair!!! They will constantly be caught playing in the locks: fluffing them unnecessarily; shaking or picking to remove imaginary dust or lint; measuring them to see if they've grown today; stroking them because it helps them think better; or just lifting them up so that they can flop back down!

As if that weren't bad enough, nobody else is able to resist the touch either!!! Friends, relatives, strangers will experience the irresistible urge to fondle and caress your locks. All will marvel at how soft they are, and how you can wear them any way you want.

Styling and grooming habits change, and overall, compared to relaxers, less time will be spent in the morning preparing for the day. And can you imagine life without a comb? no anxiety when it rains? or in the showers after a racquetball match? Women are freed up to do absolutely whatever they want, whenever they want, without hair anxieties stopping them. Sisterlocks women and Brotherlocks men become ambassadors for natural hair in the best possible way, by their example. Most are aware of being examples for others, and this also enhances their self-esteem. There is a simple miracle that I've seen occur with many of my customers: Their natural hair begins to feel simply normal to them, and this is a major milestone in their lives.

What long-term results can someone expect?

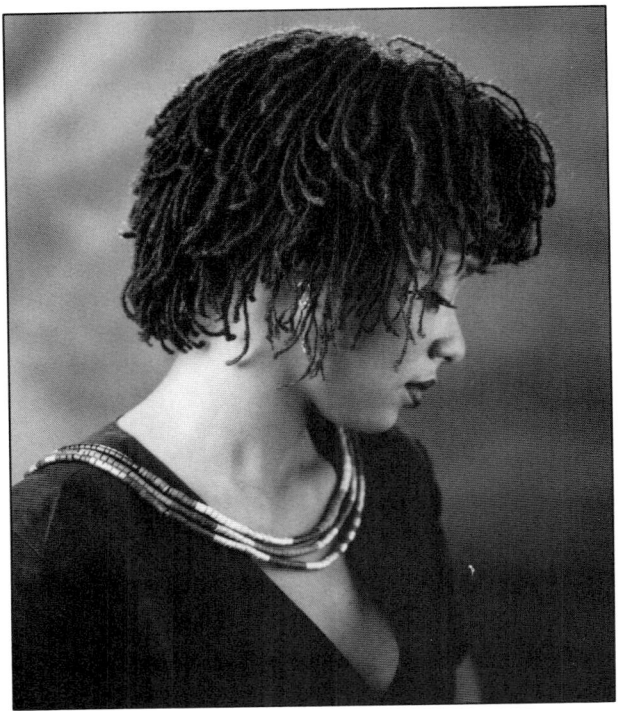

Everyone who gets Sisterlocks understands that this is not a short-term hairstyle, but a lifestyle choice they will maintain for at least several years. Maria is a good case in point. She feels she has finally found a hair system that she is comfortable with. It lets her be true to who she really is. She is a teacher, and feels that she teaches as much by her example as by the things she says to her students.

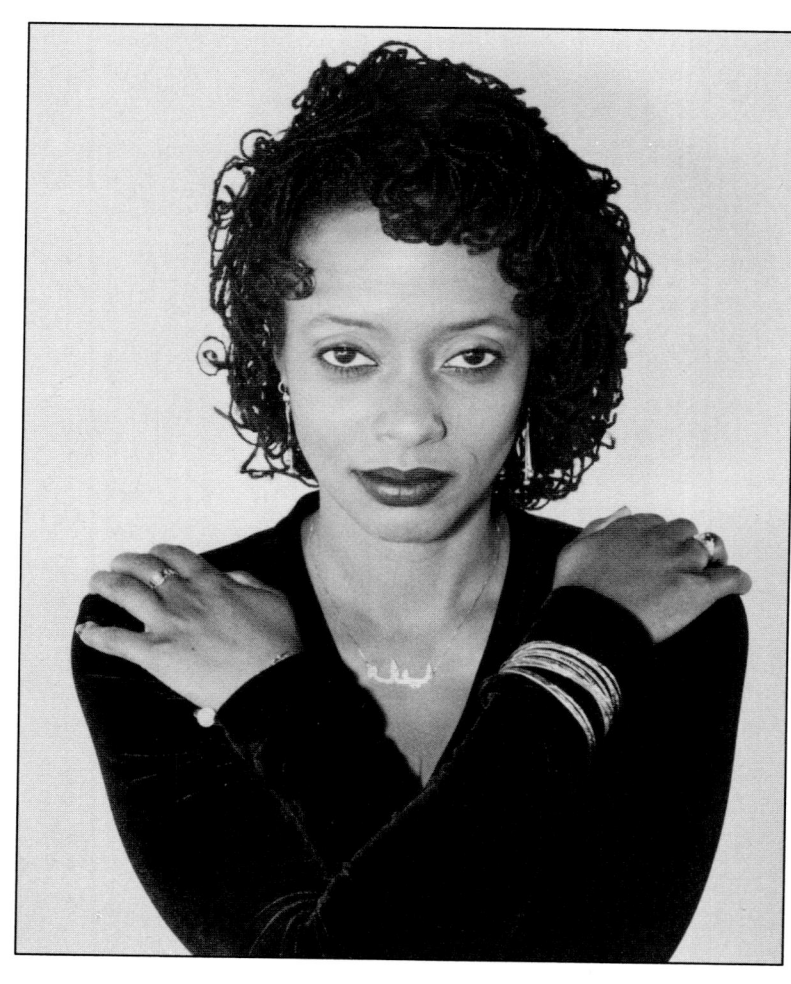

Many have the expectation that their hair will grow longer than it ever has before with Sisterlocks. Maria has found this to be the case. It took her about 2.5 years to reach her previous maximum length. She has a very thick, but fragile hair type that always broke off with relaxers. Today she is loving her new length and style.

In my case, it took about 3 years to reach my previous maximum length. As I write these words, it has been nearly 5 years, and even with my annual trimmings, my hair is still gaining length. I'm now experimenting with the limits of the durability of the locks: How long can my Sisterlocks grow and still be practical, strong and healthy? (I'll let you know.)

For the most part, our women have never been able to have the long hair they have wanted. This is of course one reason why braids have become so popular. They provide an 'ethnic' look that can have both length and style. With Sisterlocks you must grow your own length, but when the locks are properly cared for, this is not a problem. I don't believe that having the locks actually cause hair growth. More growth is simply realized because the hair is not breaking off, and the scalp is freed from the damage and stress of chemical processes or improper braiding and un-braiding techniques.

Some people express the concern that the weight of the locks will eventually put undue stress on the hair follicles, and cause the locks to break off. With my longest locks approaching 18 inches, I am not yet experiencing a heavy weight on my scalp, except when my hair is soaking wet in the shower. The weight problem may be a factor with traditional locks that can be several times more dense toward the ends than at the scalp. With mature Sisterlocks, the density along the length of the locks is very close to what it is at the scalp.

With regular grooming, it is possible to control the tendency of some hair types to bunch, and add too much density or weight to the locks.

There is only one drawback to the Sisterlocks that I have discovered: They will not style themselves! Styling versatility is after all, the main thing that sets these locks apart from other types, but you have to actually DO the styling, or they will simply hang and look like tiny, traditional locks. Many of my clients love this 'freestyle' look, and save the styling for special occasions. Others prefer to take constant advantage of the styling versatility. They have their layer cuts; they set on rollers or use pin curls or curling iron to set; they spray; they mousse; they use hair pins and clips to style and hold. Styling issues are different at every stage. Shorter hair can be shaped up with mousse without rollers or curlers; At the mid-stage, hair requires curling or rolling, but the set will stay all week; The longer the Sisterlocks get, the less tightly they will hold a curl. Coloring is an option too, as long as some careful (but easy)

> *There is only one drawback to the Sisterlocks that I have discovered: They will not style themselves!*

instructions are followed.

Sometimes I get so enthused about the Sisterlocks, I forget to tell people what they are NOT, so here goes! They are **not** braids or extensions; they are **not** a 'quick fix;' they are **not** an instant hairdo; they are **not** for people who are into neglecting their hair; they will **not** make your hair grow (you'll just keep the hair that does!); they will **not** make your hair break off or fall out; they will **not** cure dandruff, **nor** will they cause a dandruff condition to worsen; they are **not** a way to have straight-looking hair; and they will **not** cure your relationships (though they may be good therapy for this!)

I believe that soon, Sisterlocks will be a household word among those of us with naturally textured hair. There will be lots of competent consultants everywhere, available to do and maintain the locks, and teach others. There will be lots of good information about styling, coloring, you name it! Finally, we will be able to give back to our daughters something very precious - the experience of loving their lush natural hair, and ensuring that the experience of caring for it fills their lives with positive meaning.

I am not alone in feeling that Sisterlocks is helping us reclaim a healthy part of our cultural heritage that has been lost to us for a very long time. Nearly all of those I know with Sisterlocks feel the same way. I think we will be able to really celebrate the success of this natural hair care revolution when our daughters and grand daughters, at hearing about what we used to go through over our hair, will reply in disbelief, "You used to do WHAT to your hair? Why?" I look forward to that day when there will be no answer good enough for our children to accept!

PART THREE

Lock Your World:
(Testimonials and More!)

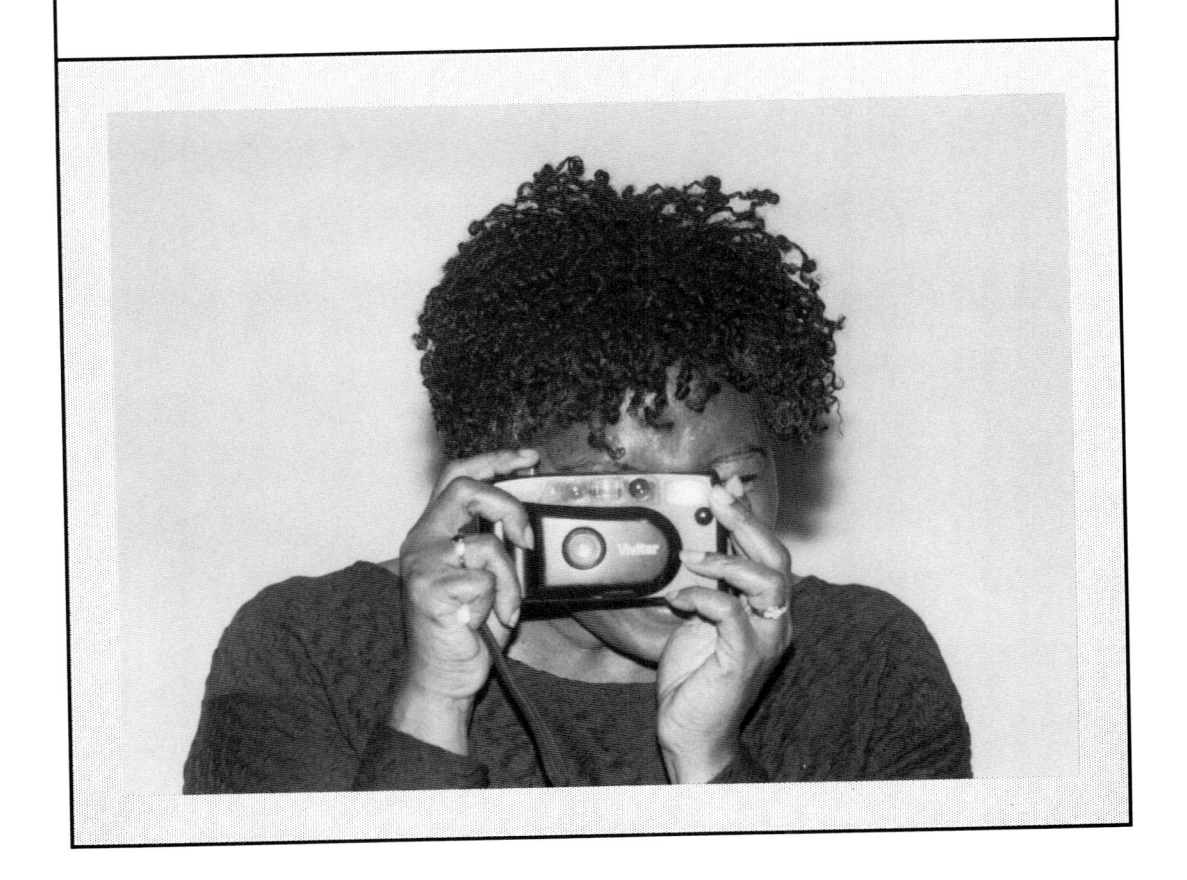

134   That Hair Thing

Jennifer

In the several years I've been doing Sisterlocks, I have found almost without exception that the decision to go with this system marks a transformational moment for our women - and men! They are coming into a deeper acceptance of themselves, and this hair styling choice becomes an outward marker of their transformation. One of the biggest rewards of doing Sisterlocks has been the chance to share in these life-transforming moments with so many people.

My customers often talk to me about what it was like for them before getting the locks, and how their lives were affected by them. None of the stories I've heard however, tops Jennifer's! All of us will be able to identify with something she says here. I think you'll agree with me: Jennifer is <u>our</u> kind of woman!

136   That Hair Thing

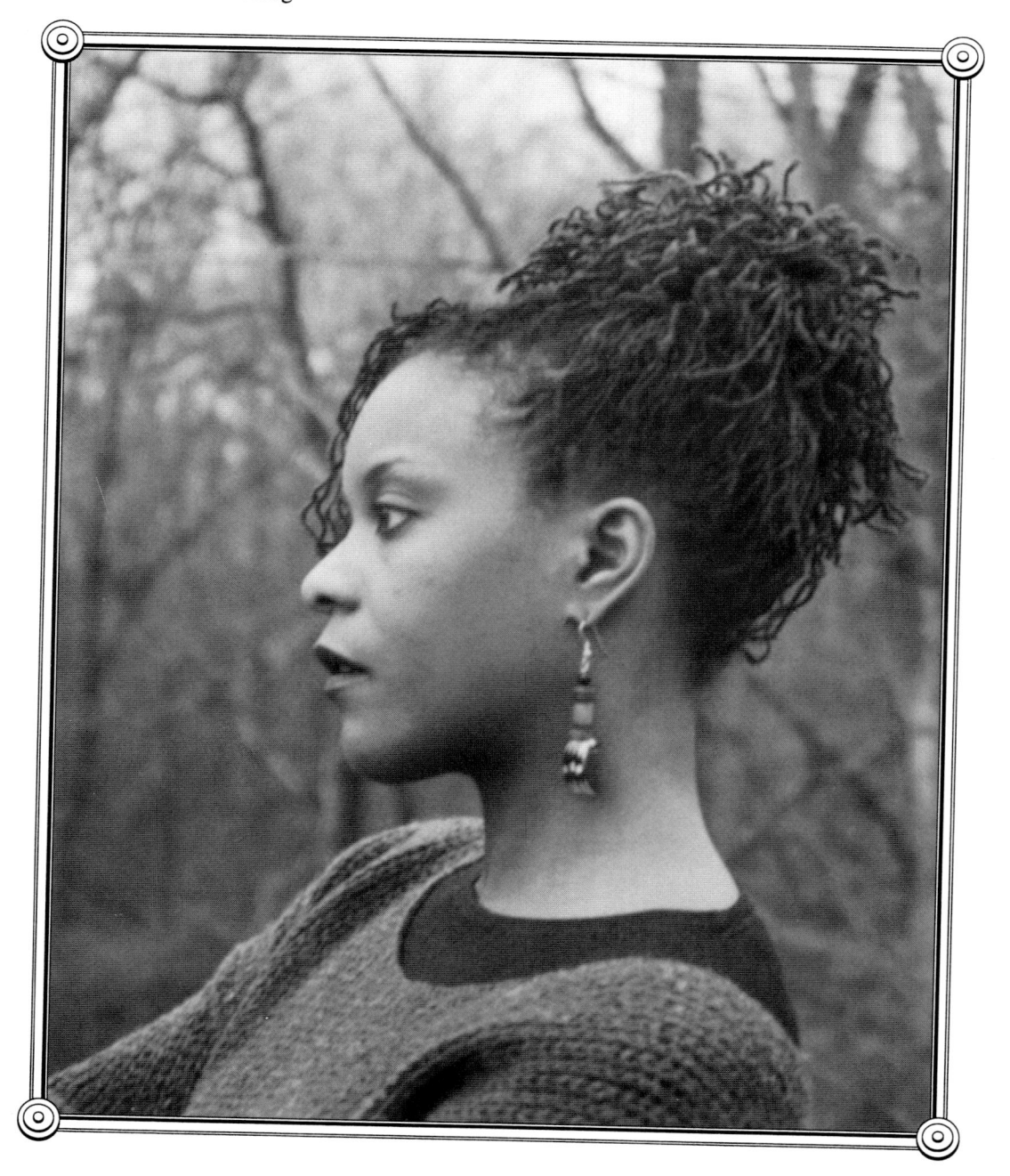

A Letter to Dr. JoAnne Cornwell from Jennifer:

Sisterlocks! *The Magic that is now my hair.*

For years, I've been looking for something to do with my hair that did not involve perming, braiding, extensions, weaving; anything artificial. Perms always destroyed my hair. At first, for about two weeks, my hair would look great. Then, my ends would split and rapidly deteriorate. Then the hair would break at the new growth. Getting a touch up only made the problem much worse. And yet, I would put my hair in thin cornrows and

> *I was so limited with what to do with my hair. No one could show me any really attractive styling options.*

extensions to get it to grow, so I could put the perm in my hair again (like a sickness!). Eventually, something like sanity began to creep in and I had to ask myself why I was putting perms in my hair. I liked length, neatness. Did I like straight? I was convinced that most men liked length and I thought I looked particularly cute with length so I stuck with the braids with extensions for years - I mean years. When I took the extensions out I noticed new growth, but the length did not last. Combing my tightly curled hair broke it off! I was so limited with what to do with my hair. No one could show me any really attractive styling options.

One salon I contacted suggested using Egyptian oil and styling gel

- then flat twist my hair and let it dry. I'd look cute for about half a day. It was greasy and sticky and I could not stand the thought of putting that stuff in my hair again for a second day. So then I'd put tiny twists in my hair and pull the back into a little bun and leave the front out for a bang. I never did leave it in long enough to lock. When I took the twists out, lots of hair came out as well. I became tired of the limited styling options for my loose, pretty, natural hair. I certainly could not wear pigtails to work, and I refused to cut it all off into a teeny, weeny Afro!

Then, when I got my March (1994) issue of Essence Magazine in the mail, I saw a small piece on Sisterlocks. Even though the photo was small, I knew this was a good idea. I did not know if it was for me, but called the number right away and got a brochure. Not good enough; I needed more information because all the brochure showed was a cute girl with her hair in little tiny locks with her hair pulled back. Nah, nah, - definitely not enough information. But it did mention that they had videos. I immediately called for the video and practically waited by the mailbox for the tape to arrive.

The first time I saw the tape I couldn't believe it so I looked at it about 15 times! I needed my hair done like this! It was very clear to me that this was finally going to be the thing that worked for my hair. Once I realized this, every day that I went without the Sisterlocks made me feel restless and uneasy. So I called the Sisterlocks office so often that they offered me the model position in Baltimore. It got canceled and I cried. They said they would have another session in Atlanta, GA and that would be two weeks away! GOD! I didn't think I could wait that long. I must have been so frantic and uptight about it, I got stomach flu with a high fever a week before it was time to go. I had my plane ticket and everything. (I really, really, really hate flying. I usually need a stiff drink to endure the take off, the journey and the landing.) My car was not working properly either, so on the way to the airport it would not go beyond 51 mph on the highway. The 45 minute drive turned into an hour and 15 minute nightmare. It took another 15 minutes to find a parking space and when I did, I ran through the airport with my luggage, a fever and severe stomach cramps to find my gate.

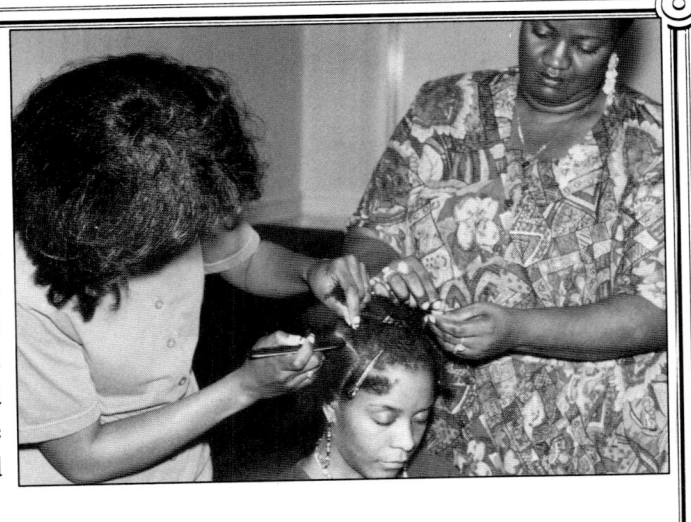

Finally, someone told me how to get to my gate but said they didn't think I would make the flight. People, you cannot imagine how much I really wanted these Sisterlocks. I was not playing! So, as out of shape and breath as I was, I ran at top speed the entire length of BWI to get my flight and I made it! When I got to the hotel in Atlanta, I saw JoAnne and it only confirmed that Sisterlocks were just gorgeous. And JoAnne looked about 5 times prettier in person. I'm sorry, but I just knew that I was going to look FINE in Sisterlocks. Two hours later, JoAnne began work on my hair.

The next day she and a number of ladies (trainees) worked on my hair and I'm not sure, but it seems it all took about 16 hours to do. It was only towards the end that I got the panic attack! "What have I done?!?" JoAnne told me that it was a normal reaction but most people got that way when the Sisterlocks were just getting put in their hair. (She also told me that even though I got the very small locks, as they began to really form, they would get fatter or expand.)

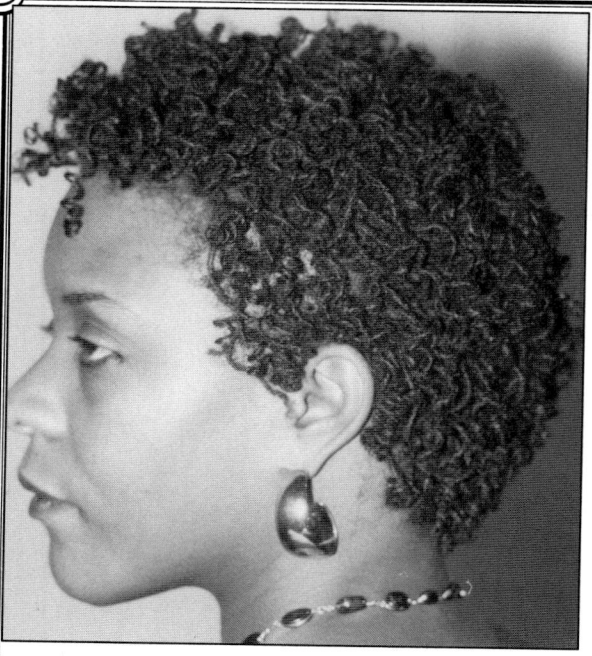

When I got home I still did not know what to do. I was given suggestions about rollers, braiding up the locks, gels and hair spray. But I had been away from styling my hair for so long that the first week or so I just pulled it back and left the bang out in front; the same thing I was tired of doing before I got the Sisterlocks. I felt bad. Did I really do this? Then my mom, whom I live with and who is my best friend, made no comment. I knew that meant she did not like them. Later we had an argument about something stupid. The day before she and I were to go to a wedding of a good friend I got the bright idea of wet setting my locks on tiny perm rods. The next day while getting dressed, my hair looked so good that it prompted my mother out of her anger and silence to tell me how good it looked. She could not wait to help me style the little curls and frame them about my face.

That day made me feel better than I had in years about my looks. At the wedding, all kinds of men were looking at me. A lady there that I would never suspect would want locks said she would like to have them. People were telling me how pretty they looked. They were putting their hands in my hair - I almost didn't know how to take this!

I wore my hair in the little curls for about a week after I first rolled them, - they last what seems to be forever when wet set in this way. And the men go wild! One day at work (and this never happens) this good looking, and I mean fine brother walked up to me and said, "I just could not sit there any longer. I just had to come ask you your name." (He was really interested but had to go talk to the auto adjuster that called him over. Rats!) Seconds later, a brother, right behind the first one came out and did the same thing. I thought they were together. They were complete strangers to each other! A co-worker who was with me at the time asked me what was going on with these guys. She was just as astounded as I was. Then she and I both realized that I wasn't giving off some scent. I just looked good!

The next week I rolled them on large rollers. All of a sudden, the fly girls at work noticed. They thought I had permed my hair. When they realized that I had not, they actually seemed very impressed. WOW! Honestly, I was really becoming more and more convinced that my Sisterlocks were magically beautiful. Not only was my hair transformed, but my personality was changing. I hadn't bought clothes in years because I had slowly begun to feel unattractive. This didn't really hit me until I had the Sisterlocks. Soon I was out shopping for clothes at lunch time at work, after work and on the weekends. (My mother was absolutely thrilled about this since she wants grandchildren so bad and I'm an only child!)

Soon, I was getting out of the house a whole lot more. I had been feeling so unattractive and I was very uncomfortable going out. It didn't used to be that way. I had felt attractive and confident wearing extension braids, though I had been a little reserved because I knew I had extensions in my hair. My hair hadn't been permed in years, and I still had not found anything to do with it that I found all that flattering. As you can imagine, I was quite miserable and was becoming quite reclusive.

It's been almost 3 months since I got my locks and I can wash them loose now. They just get prettier and more sensuous weekly. I actually feel - sexy. My friends who used to have locks told me that my formerly weak strands of hair have been made stronger by locking them, and will break at the end far less and will basically grow like weeds. They are impressed with the new technology and love my hair. I can't keep my hands out of my hair and when others touch my hair they are pleasantly surprised with how soft it is. It's so sensuous. Recently my mother confessed that when I got home with my locks, she did not like them, but now she wants them in her own hair.

I feel so good now. My hair is in its natural state and is naturally beautiful. I am so thankful to SISTERLOCKS for positively changing my life. It's been a cathartic experience, an adventure of love and beauty that will only get better and better. I love it!

(April, 1994)

Jennifer has gone on to become trained in the Sisterlocks system. Today she is a Certified Consultant, and hopes to become a Certified Training Associate, so that she can teach Sisterlocks. She is the kind of dedicated individual who will help us carry Sisterlocks to the next level!

When I asked Jennifer what her life has been like in the three years since she wrote us this letter, she replied:

"It's just gotten better! Now and again I'll freak out momentarily over being the 'only one' with this look. Over all though, I'm not as keen on the validation as I thought I'd be. Most of the time I forget I have this unique look, and wonder why I'm getting so much attention!"

"It's neat to get so many compliments out of the blue from so many different kinds of people. It's been great fun, but also, it opens you up to self-appreciation!"

Blinded By The Light

Dennard Clendenin has worked with the Sisterlocks team since day-one. He is a steadfast supporter of the concept, and has remained in the trenches with us through thick and thin. When I asked him to contribute something to this work from a male perspective, true to form, he got right on it. When I read what he produced I was blown away! I really got more than I bargained for.

His honesty is at times troubling, but it brings to light the inner turmoil many of our men go through, and explains how this can affect how they relate to us. After reading this, I think you will see why Dennard has earned the affectionate title of the Sisterlocks Brother.

144   That Hair Thing

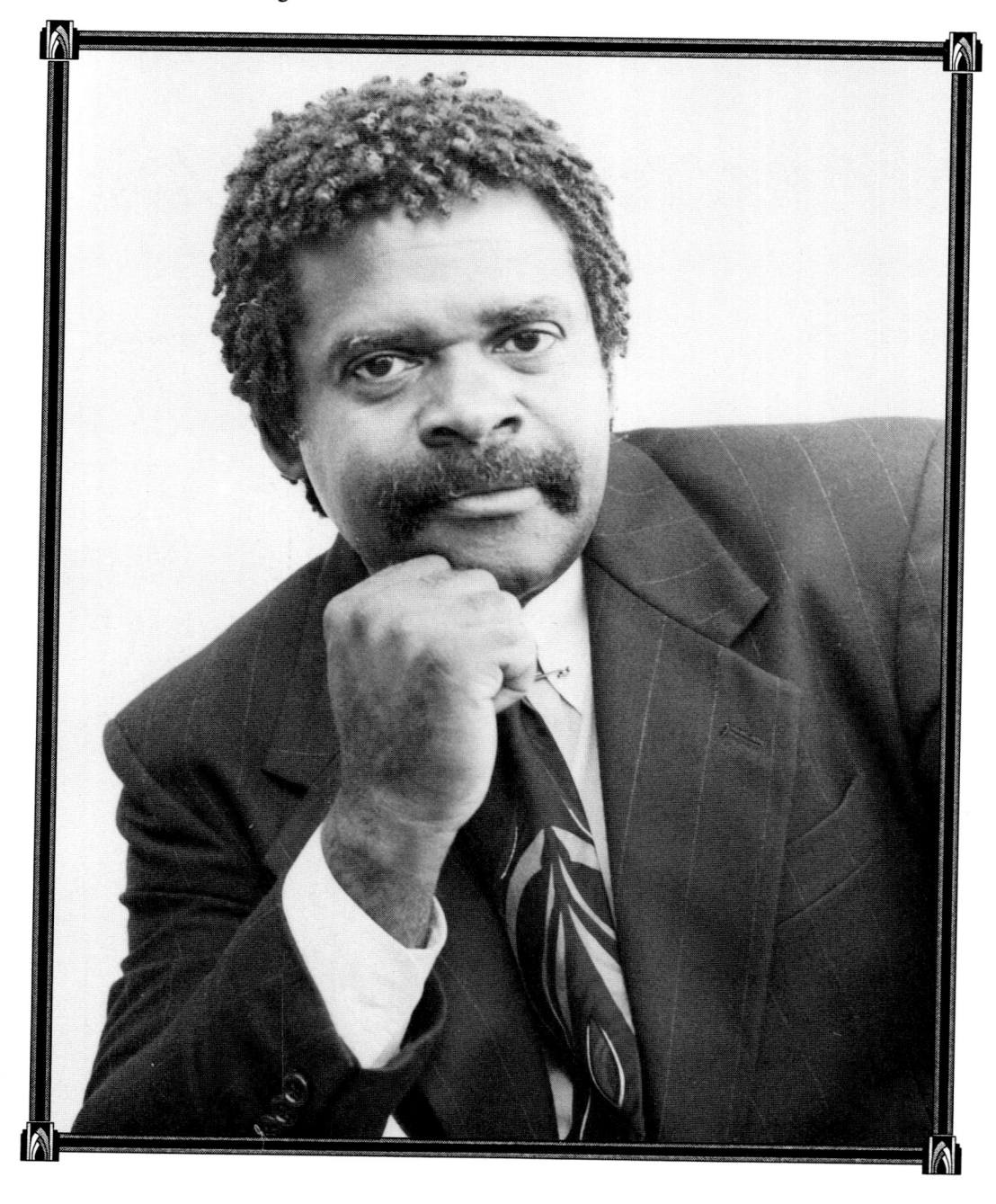

Blinded by the Light
by
Dennard Clendenin

I do not remember meeting my mother until I was fourteen years old, and my father, some fourteen years after that. You might say my situation typified what Daniel Patrick Moynihan characterized as "...The tangled web of social pathology...," as it dealt with the black family in America. As it turned out, I had the good fortune to be raised by my grandmother, who was my rock, protector, provider, mother, father, and Santa Claus all in one. In addition to her, my aunt and sister were ever present. As an African American male, I consider myself blessed to have come from such wonderful, matriarchal beginnings. Why, then, I wondered was I motivated to seek personal relationships with white women?

At one point in my life, I was totally absorbed with the prospect of finding and securing a white mate. You might say I was "blinded by the light.." It really didn't matter to me whether the woman was attractive, wealthy, or even feminine; it was her white skin and, yes, blonde hair that mattered most. Why did I feel the need to reject black women, considering the loving and nurturing environment provided for me by the women in my own family?

If we look historically at male/female dynamics, women have always been one of the significant spoils of war; possessions passed from vanquished to victor. I propose that these dynamics are still at work today. They manifest themselves during armed conflict, as evidenced in the Bosnian War. Since men can be victimized by other men through the abuse of their women, it adds to the sense that she is less a person than a possession to be won, hidden and used when it is to the man's advantage.

Also, men still choose women based on what comes along with the "package;" like status, or material wealth. Add to this the images of women in general, and white women in particular that permeate our media, and we can see why the image of her as the ideal 'possession' remains so strong.

I know that it is popular to blame the media for events that occur in our lives, and I want to assure you that this is not a media witch hunt. But consider the proliferation of white women in the media during my upbringing in the fifties and sixties. Although kitchen appliances and automobiles were hawked by the ubiquitous male voice over, it was the image of the white female that really sold the soap. The same image was replicated in cigarette, liquor, and travel ads. For me, as for many like me, a message was implanted that in order to succeed, I needed to have a white woman. Even the Mickey Mouse Club, through the person of Annette Funicello with her pixie smile and budding breasts, had a hand in providing many a sexual fantasy for just about every prepubescent boy in America. Annette was the topic of conversation in our "boys only" clubs, cafeterias, gym locker rooms, school yards and scribbling on restroom walls. And although we may not admit it, this image was the vehicle through which many of us discovered and indeed explored our bodies.

Playboy and other magazines had us swooning over pictures of such blonds as Marilyn Monroe and Jayne Mansfield; Kim Novak and Edie Adams ("The minute you walked in the joint, I could see you were a man of distinction..."). Then there was our hero, Sammy Davis Jr., who had the Swedish blond bombshell, May Britt. I was never exposed to the sensuality or sultriness of our own beauties like Lena Horne, Dorothy Dandridge or Josephine Baker. Cicily Tyson and Abby Lincoln did get a little play, but most of the black women I saw on the screen were more like Butterfly McQueen and Hattie McDaniel. Today I understand that these women did their best with the limited roles they were dealt. In fact, because of them, later actresses would have choices that were less demeaning. But when I was a youth, all I knew was that women on the screen who looked like us held no attraction for me whatsoever!

And this scenario has not completely disappeared. Increasingly, black athletes and celebrities are found to be part of interracial relationships. I believe that this sends the same "spoils of war" message to young black males who live their lives in terms of athletic success and the so-called rewards that go with it. Partly as a result of messages like these, I concluded that with a white woman on my arm I could gain access to those luxuries I never saw associated with black women. In other words, while I equated black women with strength (not necessarily considered a favorable trait in a woman) I equated white women with power. (Witness the fact that there is very little power attributed to black women, thus we offer the backhanded compliment of calling them "strong.") I believe that these messages greatly influenced my preference and ultimate marriage to a white woman. Although I believe that I loved my wife, I now know there was a great deal of dissonance for me, throughout our relationship.

I freely admit that at one time dark skin and 'nappy' hair were anathema for me. I saw no social advantage or redeeming qualities to "looking like that." Prior to the television show "Julia," depicting a single parent-head of household (no black man) in the 1960s, black women were portrayed as overweight, domineering, and non-sexual beings. Of course growing up in the 50s, I never associated my grandmother, aunt, or sister with sexuality of any sort, but white girls would really stop me in my tracks! I could be having a conversation with a black girl, and if a white one walked by, I would literally stop my conversation and stare. I remember pining over Kathy K., and ignoring Linda H., Cynthia L., or Joyce J. I even recall watching the Miss Black America Pageant, in the early seventies and labeling them "all ugly." On several occasions my insensitivity towards black women was challenged by the sisters themselves. Mary C. provided me with a very blunt and painful retort one evening when she stated, "You can't handle a black woman!" For me it was a rude awakening, as well as the truth.

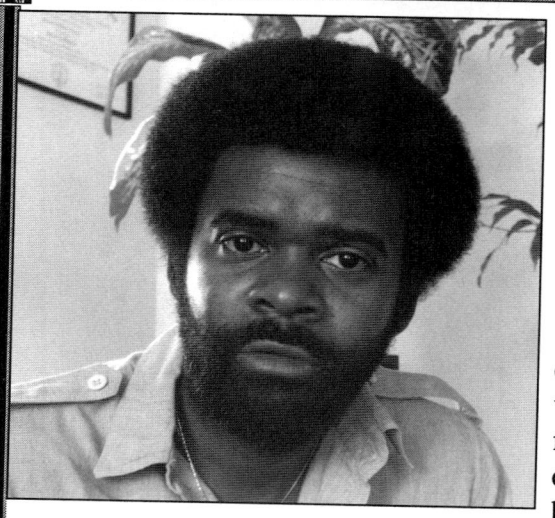

It was shortly after my divorce, that the pendulum swung in the other direction. I started seeking the exclusive company of black women. However, she had to be a "certain kind of black woman." I also remember quite vividly, expecting them to act like white women. I wanted them to take my stuff without question. I expected them to have "good hair." If I found myself with someone who wore an afro, though I wore one myself, I felt strange and had to force myself to relax. I imagined that she was manly, and probably bossy. I also found myself gravitating towards lighter skinned women. I was caught up in my own pathology! Unfortunately, I think that the preferences I showed then are still evident in young black men today, if the rap videos featuring almost exclusively light skinned women with wavy hair are any indication.

I have to say that my own reeducation was helped along through my work as part of the Sisterlocks team. I saw first hand, the metamorphosis in clients as they became beautiful, largely as a result of coming to a new way of feeling about themselves. I witnessed moments that seemed magical to me, when several women in a room would be focused on each others hair, not talking, just helping each other connect with something they all seemed to know had been there the whole time. They loved themselves, and you could see it in their faces. Shooting their pictures also gave me the opportunity to pay attention to them as I never had before. I felt as though I was being brought to consciousness. Their hair textures especially intrigued me. This is amazing, I thought! Why hadn't I seen this before!

When I decided to get locked myself, I never dreamed that the metamorphosis I saw in women would descend on me. I feel my hair now, and I love to touch it. You couldn't touch your afro, and you'd mess it up if you ran your fingers through it. My locks draw silent looks of affirmation from other men, especially those who are also locked. Young kids are taken by it and want to know how they can get it. I've even been stopped on the highway by a brother who just had to know where he could get his hair done like mine. And the women just love it. All women. And they want to touch it too. I also love the process of getting my hair re-tightened. I've never experienced that kind of thing before. There is something primal about it, like a bonding experience. It always puts me to sleep.

Today, I like to say that I was lost and now I am found. I am no longer blinded by the light. I love African descended women with all of their unique features, but especially their hair. I love kinky/nappy hair. Playing with my partners long natural locks gives me a great deal of pleasure. I keep my hands in her hair almost to a distraction. I have no desire to run my fingers through RIO. If I see a sister who is fine, but her hair is "treated," it diminishes her beauty for me. I made a decision never to seek partnerships with women who smoke. It's unhealthy. As a result of my reeducation and appreciation for our natural hair, I have also decided to never seek relationships with women who are not comfortable with their hair. It's unhealthy. I realize that one should never say never, however for me it is a matter of choice. It is very unlikely that I will compromise this value. I choose to be with a life partner who is steeped in her natural beauty.

That Hair Thing

Men On Hair

I used to think that hair issues only concerned women. Boy, was I mistaken! I've learned that most men are very concerned about their hair as it relates to their overall appearance, <u>and</u> their sense of identity. Not only this, but the question about natural vs. processed hair is also a big one for many of them too, and for many of the same reasons as for us women.

I've asked some of our Brotherlocks men to comment on these things. I think you'll agree with me after reading these pages, that we'll gain the most when we come together over this hair thing!

Name:

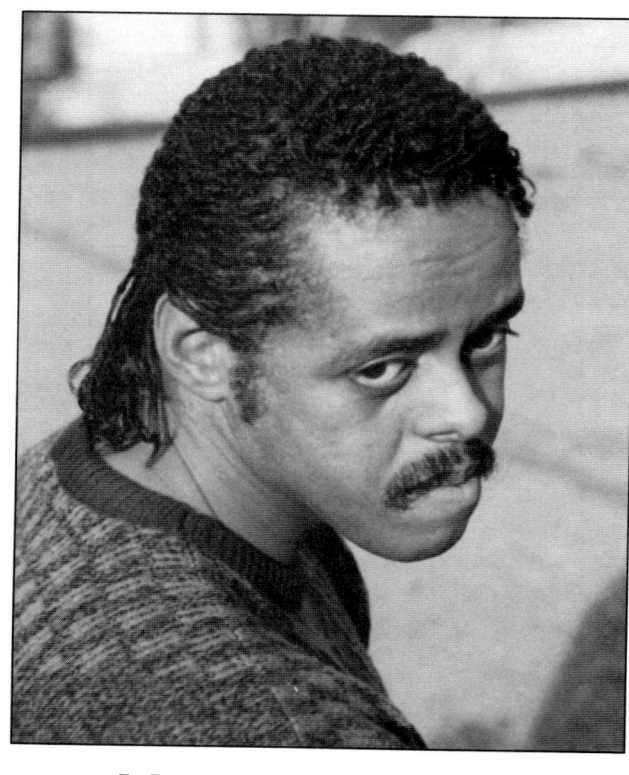

Michael

Occupation:

Hotel Maintenance

Time in Locks: 3 years

Michael is a soft spoken kind of guy. He doesn't complain about much, and he's not the demanding type. Who would have thought that Michael was going through life, hating his hair and feeling self-conscious about his looks!

Women tend to think that **we** have all the good-hair, bad-hair issues, but Michael can tell you what it's like for a guy with hair that has a very tight natural texture.

Michael has tried nearly every conceivable product and process, in an effort to get the look he felt most comfortable with. Little did he know all those years that he had absolutely ideal hair for locking! "I don't have to put anything in my hair, and it shines on its own. Now I look at all those relaxers and waves and stuff, and ask myself 'why'?"

When asked how having the locks has affected his job, Michael smiled and replied, "It's made life easier. I can sleep longer now before work!" "People at work are curious. They ask a lot of questions. Some thought they were extensions. Most people like it."

Because of all the things he's gone through over his own hair, Michael is really attuned to what we women go through. Though he loves his own locks, he tries not to judge what women do to their hair. He says he likes <u>all</u> types of looks on women, as long as their hair is well taken care of.

Name: **Ernie**

Occupation: Engineer

Time in Locks: 1 year

"When we concede to looking the way other people think we should look, we keep them comfortable in their control over us."

Ernie has thought a lot about natural hair and locks, and what they mean to people. "As long as you're unaware, there's no problem" he says. "But once you become aware and see the impact of this, it really hurts your feelings!"

When Ernie decided to get locked himself, he confronted his uneasiness about how this might affect his job by talking directly with his boss. "He didn't have a problem with it. Now, not a week goes by that I don't get compliments. Mostly from whites." "This is something we have that is uniquely African!"

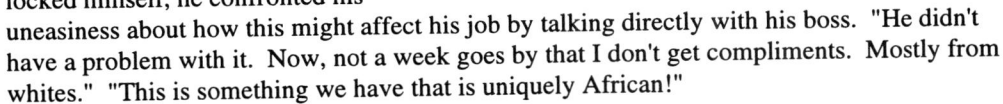

Though the vast majority of people Ernie encounters are accepting of his locks, it has been suggested off the record that they could get in the way of another promotion for him. When asked how he would react if this turned out to be true, Ernie replied, "I would never cut my locks for this reason. We don't want to feed white supremacy. Besides, it could be a blessing in disguise - a push for me to become more independent."

Ernie says he's breaking the mold so that the next brother who wants to get locks won't have to deal with the various stereotypes he has had to deal with. "We have a unique kind of beauty," he reminds us. "We should be proud of it!"

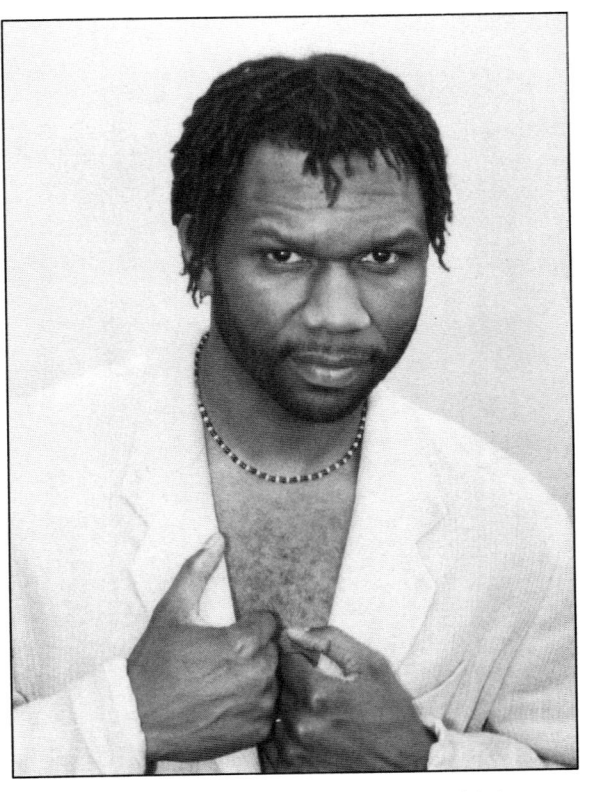

Name:

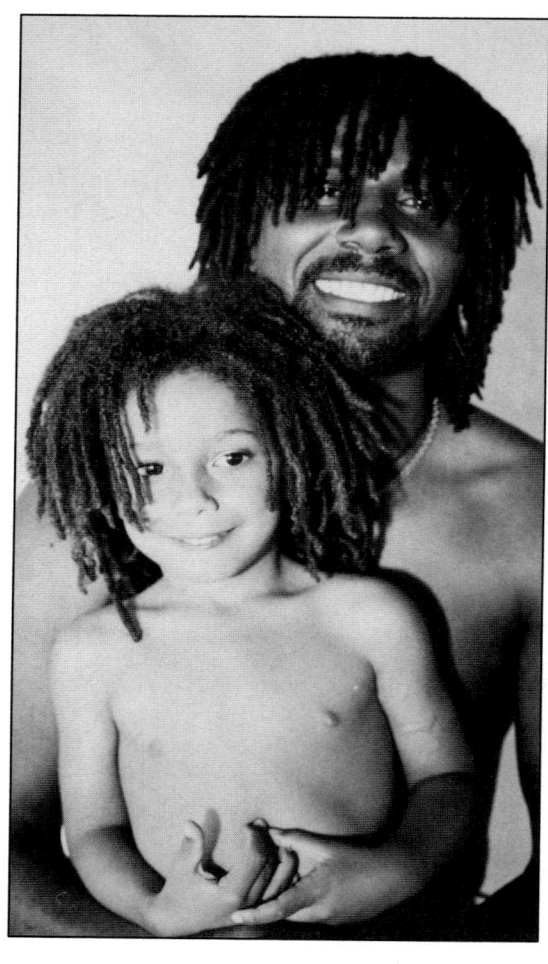

Ed

Occupation:

Business Owner

Time in Locks: 1 year

Locks seemed to be a natural for Ed's young son. Some friends reacted in shock though, saying that was an outlandish idea. "It's nothing I wouldn't do for myself," replied Ed, and proved it by getting locks himself. Little did he know that he would truly fall in love with them.

Ed has experimented with a lot of different hair treatments. In high school he wore a big, really big Afro. Next it was the relaxer/roller routine. For a time, that was "cool", but in the back of his mind he wasn't really satisfied. The curl came next, but that was too greasy on the shirt collars. Then came the short, neatly manicured military look. After a while, Ed's busy lifestyle couldn't accommodate those frequent trips to the barber.

Today, he likes the freedom and uniqueness of his locks. "They make me feel more me," he says. They definately make the right statement for Ed. "There are a lot of expectations on Black men, expecially in the business world." "I'm not big on conformity!"

Ed has what he wants, and does fine with the mixed reactions he gets. Typically, the positive comments about his hair do NOT come from African Americans, who tend to just look and say nothing. What about Ed's son? Well, he thinks his dad is really COOL!

Name:
Dawud

Occupation:

Business Owner / Employee Coordinator for Clothing Company

Time in Locks:
2.5 years

Working part time in the corporate world and part time in his personal business, Dawud's high profile lifestyle keeps him in contact with lots of people. A rogue at heart, he originally wanted to create a look that he knew would NOT be acceptable in corporate America. His locks turned out to have exactly the opposite effect however! He gets compliments daily, and is seen by colleagues as an innovator and someone with extra confidence.

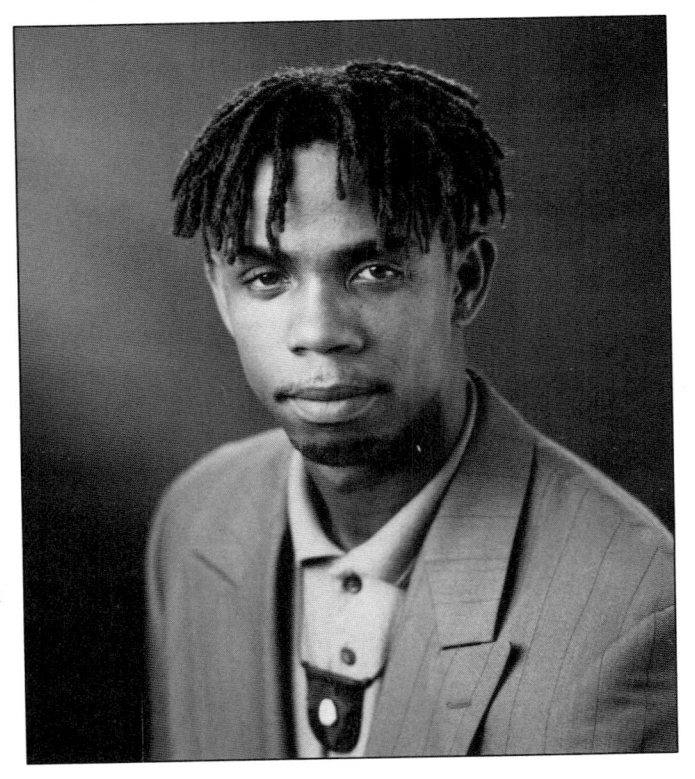

"This is it." he asserts. "I can't imagine myself without locks. It's caused so many positive changes in my life. " One case in point is when Dawud finds himself around other black men. He feels that his hair causes a breakdown of a kind of wall of fear that has prevented our men from opening up to each other. This is especially true of younger men in the 18 - 21 age group who now seem more culturally conscious.

Perhaps the best thing about his locks is that Dawud regularly gets mistaken for someone on TV. "At least once a week I get asked if I'm some actor on a sitcom, or a US world cup soccer player. I really don't mind! Once though, a woman swore I was wearing a weave. It didn't matter what I said or did, she would not be convinced that this is my real hair." Dawud knows that you can't win them all, but you can bet that he's winning the ones that count!

That Hair Thing

Name: James

Occupation: Film and Video Editor

Time in Locks: 2 years

You'd think living in LA, a guy could get exactly what he wanted done to his hair! Not so for James who searched high and low before finding the Brotherlocks he now loves. "With my work, locks are no problem. Lots of things are considered normal."

James has been a trend setter his whole life. He's never felt bound by any style, and locks are no exception. As natural as they feel for him though, he says he probably won't keep them forever. "They're not a big political thing for me. I just followed the natural process of things."

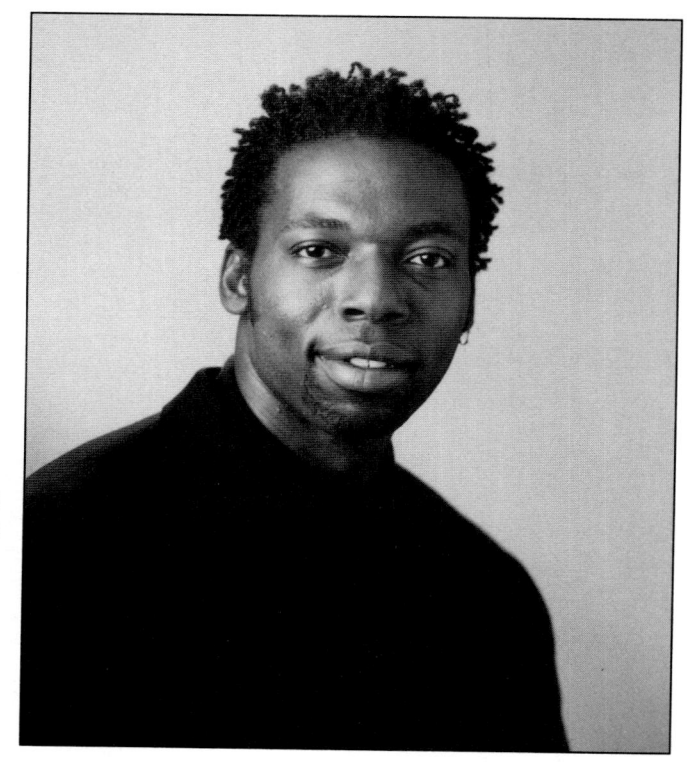

According to James, someone's hair choices should be seen as irrelavent to their ability to perform. Natural or processed, one shouldn't be seen as better than the other. Anyway, it's all relative, as his travels to Europe confirm. In France and England his hair is admired, but in Germany, Italy and Switzerland, people really "freak out." "People stare. I'm seen as an oddity." The exception to this is among the younger set. "Kids everywhere just love my hair. They admire African Americans because we're strong and we take chances. To actually see one of us with locks just confirms what they've imagined."

Says James, "The world is not quite ready for African Americans. They don't know how to take us." James is helping to change this, and for the moment he may feel out there on his own. But hang on! There are millions more of us, and we're not far behind!

Name: Keith

Occupation: Security Investigations

Time in Locks: 2 years

Some people identify really closely with their hair and some people don't. Keith definately derives a deep sense of identity from his natural locks. "I just feel blacker! This is mine! This is ours!" Keith has always been conscious of what hair represents, and now more than ever, he wears his as a badge.

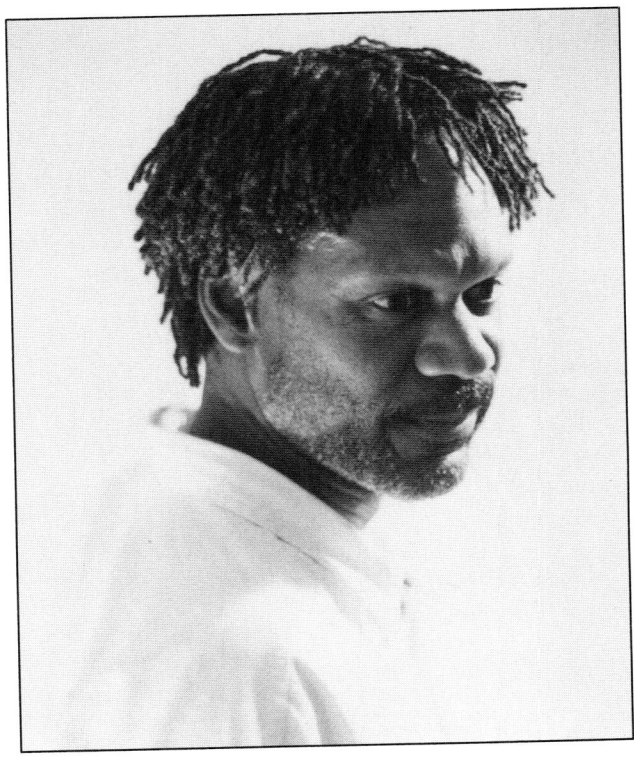

Keith finds symmetry in the unruliness of his locks. This reminds him of his own personality. "I'm a wild guy anyway. My hair goes all different ways and so do I." A risk taker at heart, he loves the fact that his hair makes him stand out. Curioiusly though, this has had a very positive effect. Because of his height (6'6") his deep voice and sharp features, Keith has always made an intimidating first impression on people. With locks that has all changed. He finds people now feel comfortable approaching him. His locks give people a reason to make conversation with him. "This has never happened to me before. It really gives me a heightened feeling of acceptance."

Keith admits that he rarely talks to other black men about hair. "It's not a guy thing" he asserts. Despite their silence on the subject, they can't take their eyes off Keith's hair. "We could be talking about anything, but all the while they're looking at my hair. It's like they're talking to my hair!" Unlike many men, Keith has always liked natural hair on women. Braids, Afros or what have you. "I appreciate a woman like that!"

That Hair Thing

Name: David

Occupation: Merchant Marine

Time in Locks: 9 months

David is a meticulous kind of guy. During the '70s he liked his Afro just so. During the '80s he tried the chemical look, but it never quite gave him what he wanted. Today David is locked, and just as meticulous as ever.

In fact, he says he's more conscious than ever of both his own hair and others' hair. He believes it's because of the freedom of that comes with having locks. He likes the low maintenance. "Just keep 'em clean and let 'em go."

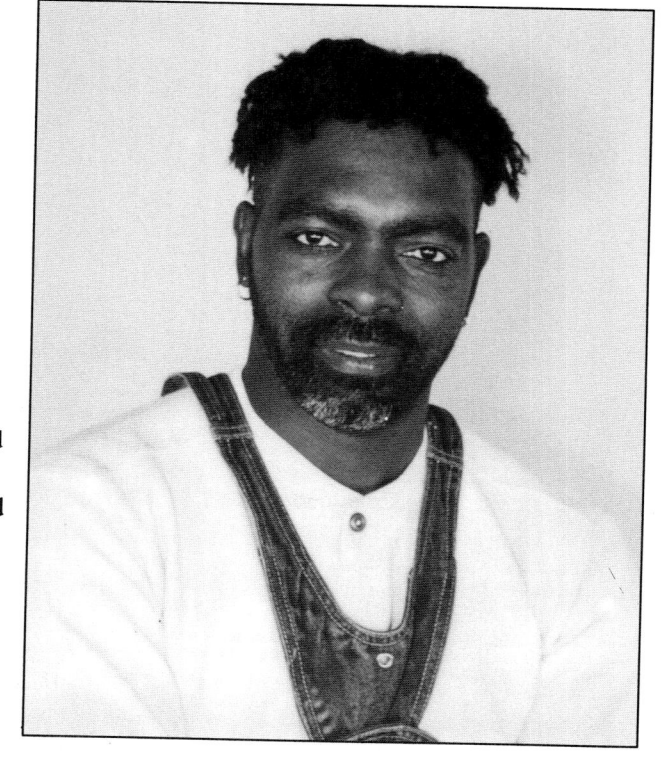

Getting his locks through the settling-in phase was somewhat of a challenge for David, who loves to scrub around wildly in his hair when he washes it. With that phase behind him though, he's in his element. Working as a merchant marine keeps David in a fairly conservative environment, yet he's had no negative reactions to his hair. "As long as I can get the fire fighting mask and hood over my head and face, they can't say a thing to me!" Some of his co-workers in fact, seem to have a stake in his new natural look. THEY remind HIM when it's time to go in for his re-tightening!

Today David still knows what he likes, and he'll tell you in a minute. "Get rid of those perms and chemicals." They're bad for you, he says, and true to form, he has a collection of articles to back up his point. "Go back to your own natural hair. Be kinky!"

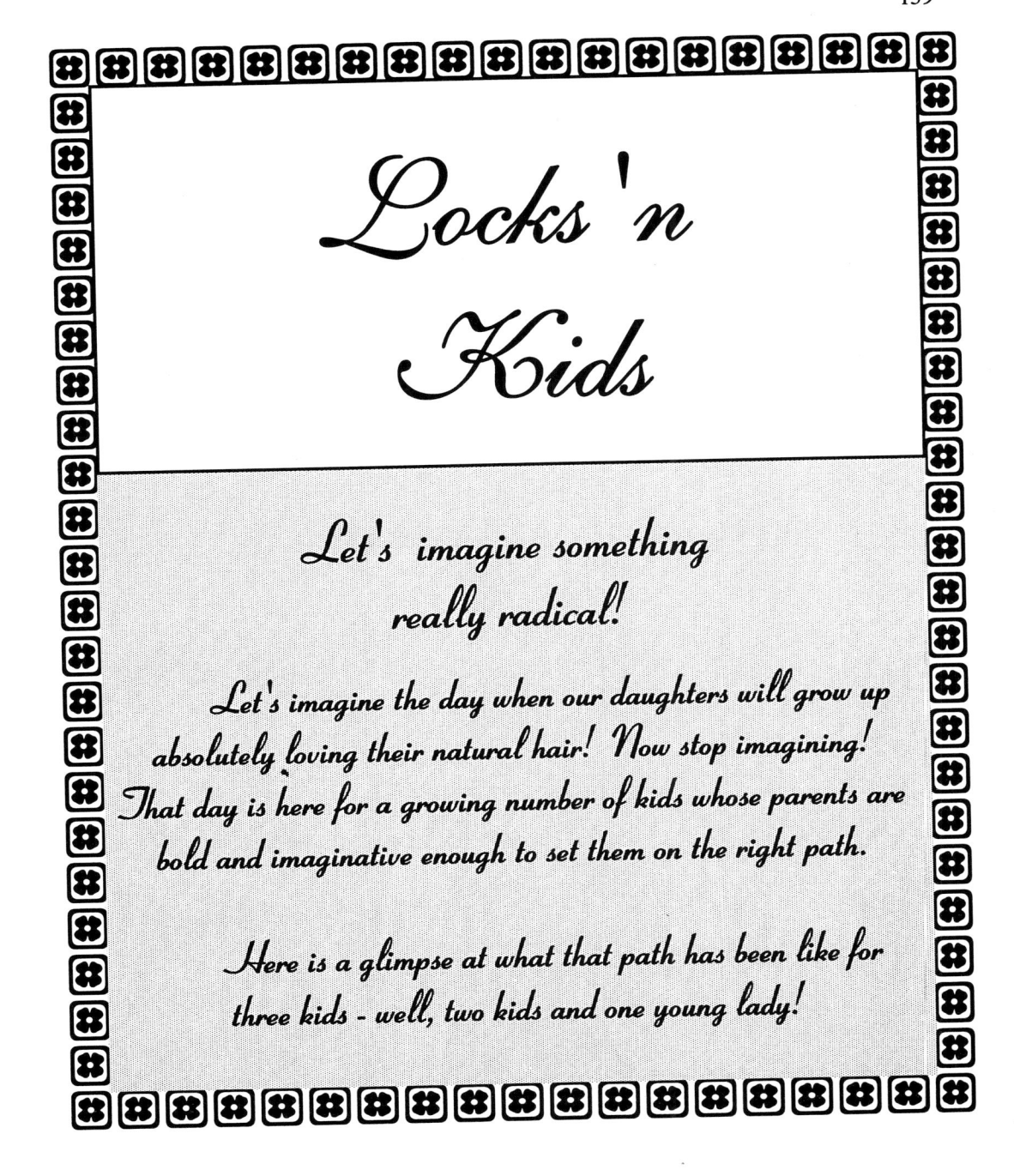

Locks 'n Kids

Let's imagine something really radical!

Let's imagine the day when our daughters will grow up absolutely loving their natural hair! Now stop imagining! That day is here for a growing number of kids whose parents are bold and imaginative enough to set them on the right path.

Here is a glimpse at what that path has been like for three kids - well, two kids and one young lady!

Giovannie - 11

JC: Whose idea was it for your daughter to get locks?
Sylvia: Both of ours. I wanted to stop combing and braiding, and she wanted something different from the braids.

JC: Giovannie, what made you want locks?
Giovannie: They grow so long and pretty, and you stick out from all the rest. You feel really proud when you have them.

JC: You're not afraid to be different?
Giovannie: Not afraid at all!

JC: What do the other kids say?
Giovannie: Sometimes they just come up to me and start playing with my hair and say it's really neat! The people who are jealous call me names. Mostly boys. I really don't care about them. Some of the girls who wear braids and stuff, you know that they really don't like their hair.

JC: Do you like your hair?
Giovannie: I love it. It's fun and different. You don't have to look like everybody else!

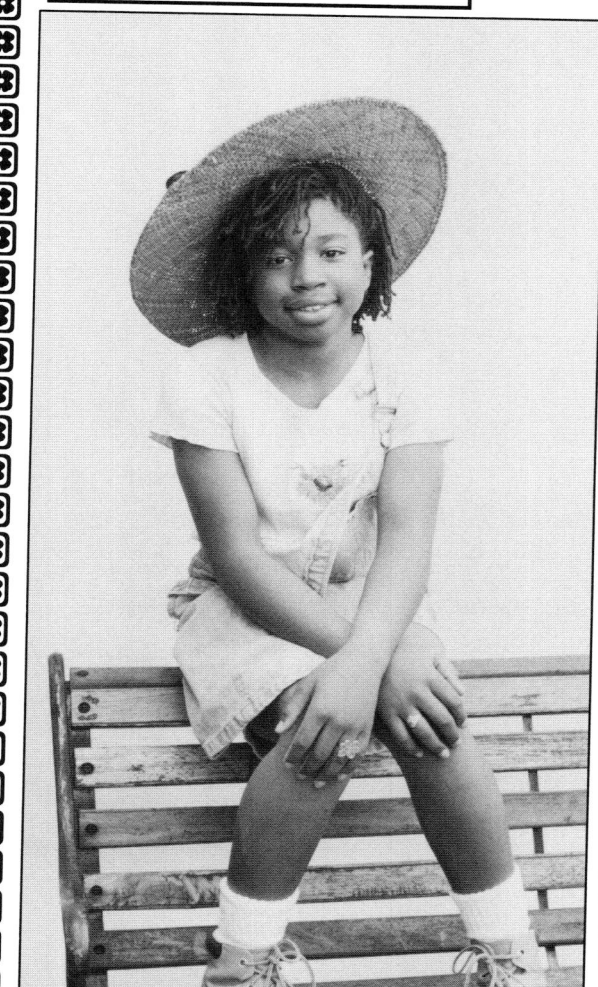

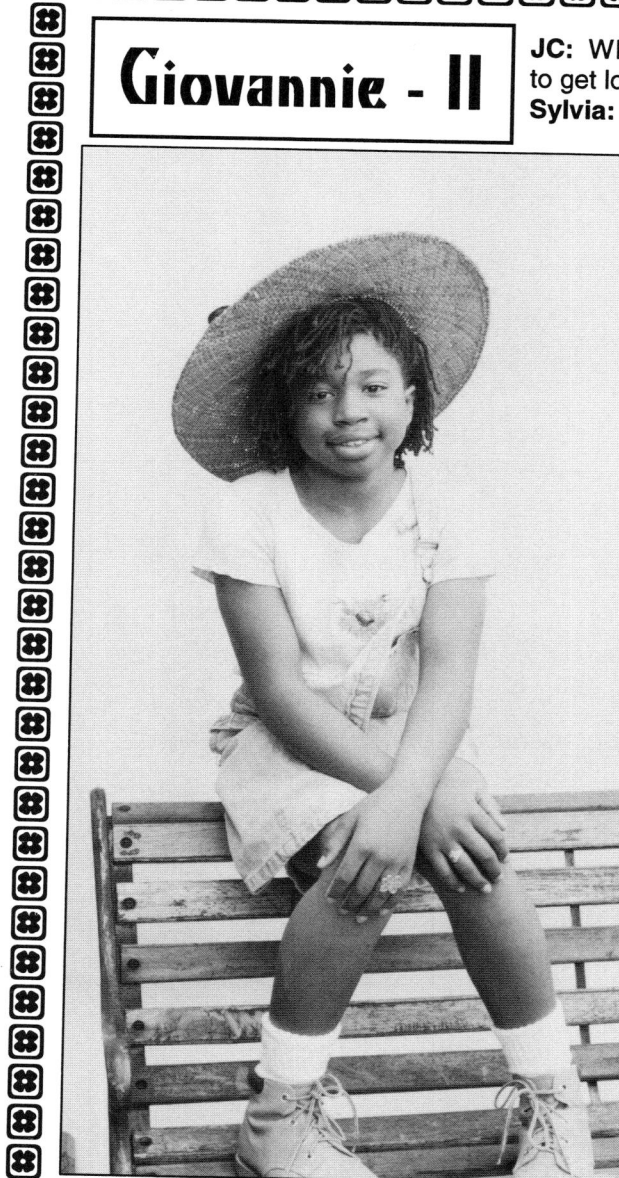

Shani - 6

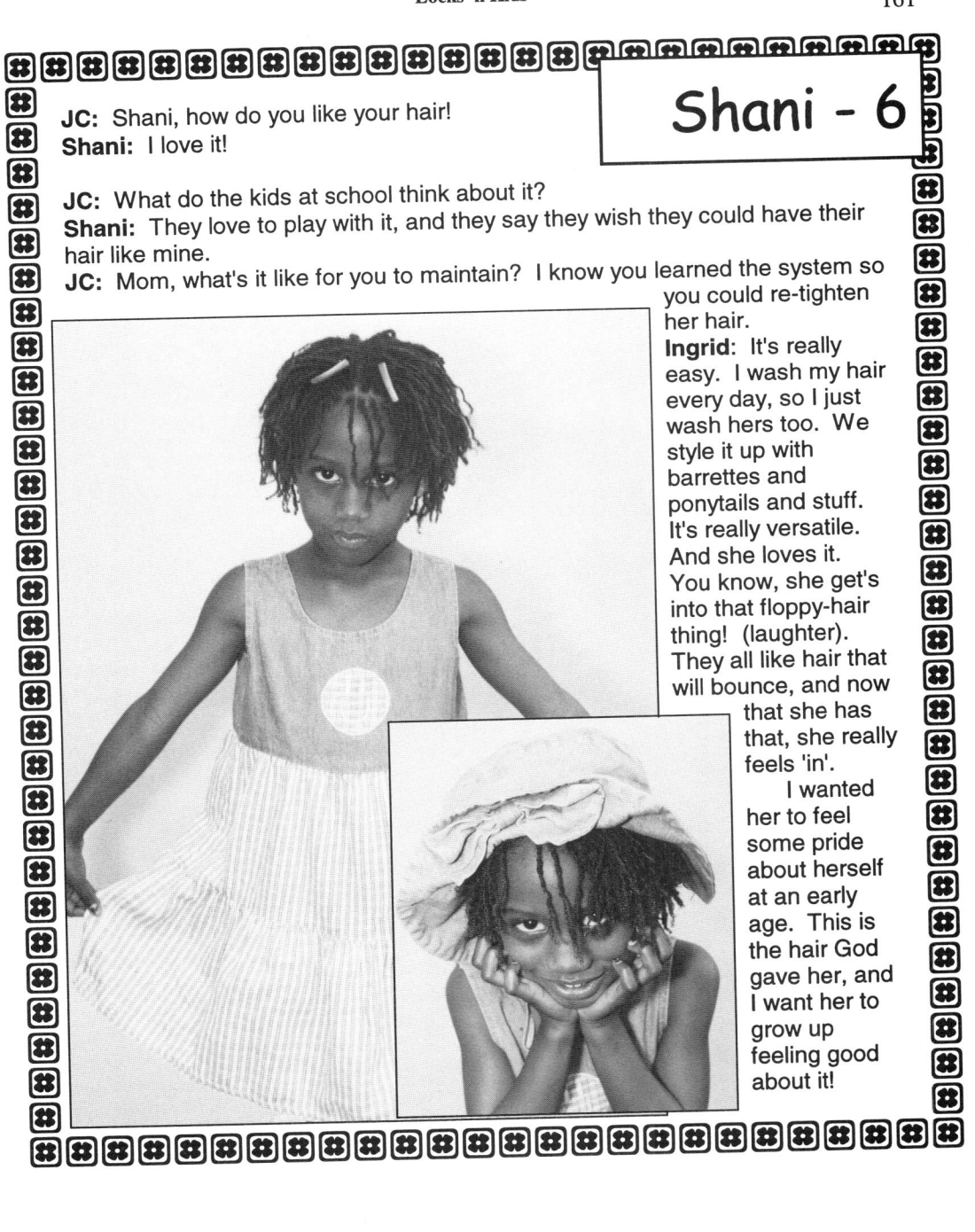

JC: Shani, how do you like your hair!
Shani: I love it!

JC: What do the kids at school think about it?
Shani: They love to play with it, and they say they wish they could have their hair like mine.

JC: Mom, what's it like for you to maintain? I know you learned the system so you could re-tighten her hair.

Ingrid: It's really easy. I wash my hair every day, so I just wash hers too. We style it up with barrettes and ponytails and stuff. It's really versatile. And she loves it. You know, she get's into that floppy-hair thing! (laughter). They all like hair that will bounce, and now that she has that, she really feels 'in'.

I wanted her to feel some pride about herself at an early age. This is the hair God gave her, and I want her to grow up feeling good about it!

Etosha - 16

JC: Mom, was it your idea to get Etosha into locks?
Anne: Not really. She was all for it. She was tired of chemicals, and didn't enjoy getting her hair pressed. I didn't have to talk her into it.
JC: Etosha, your mom tells me you've always been really confident, and that your natural locks just bring that out in you more.
Etosha: Yeah. It makes you feel really liberated. No all-day salons, and no chemicals on your head. I can go to a pool, and do lots of stuff to it. I have a lot more choices. With a curl I was always afraid of people touching my hair. It was so greasy. This is really easy to manage.

JC: Your hair has grown a lot since you've had locks.

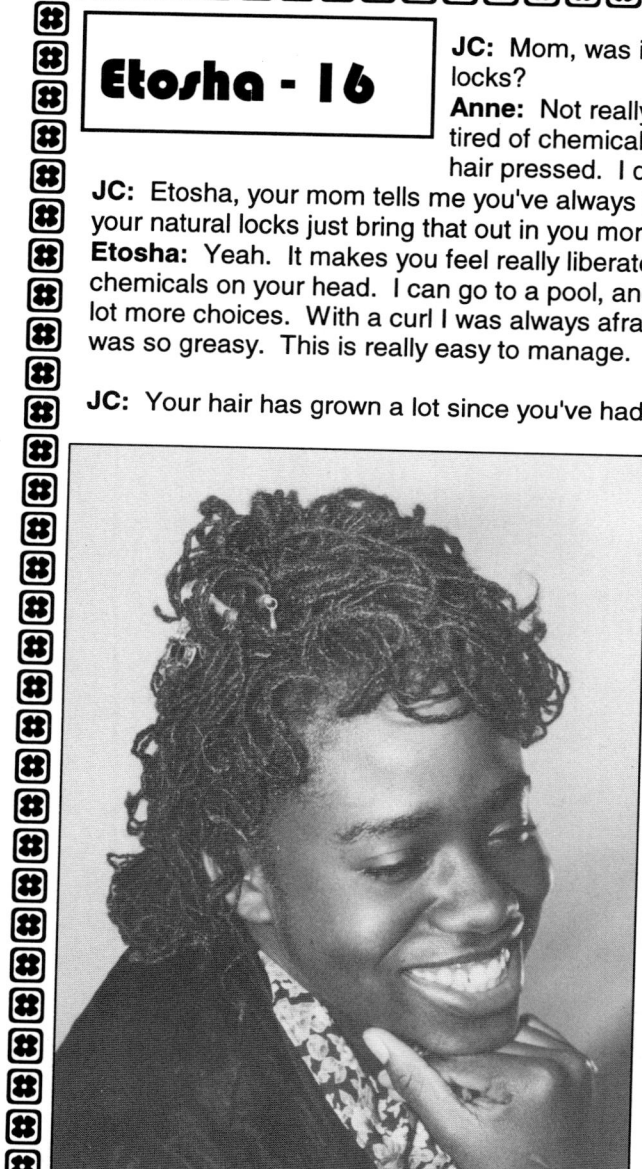

Etosha: Yeah! I think that's great!
JC: What do your peers think about it?
Etosha: My close friends are use to me now. It's just a part of me. The new people ask a lot of questions.
JC: How do the other young ladies wear their hair?
Etosha: Weaves, processed, relaxed. I don't like to judge, but they seem a little closed minded. They look at the girls in the music videos and stuff. The fad is more for them.
JC: What would you say to someone like this?
Etosha: Don't be afraid! If anything, it'll help a person out. It's much easier. I'd sure do it all over again!

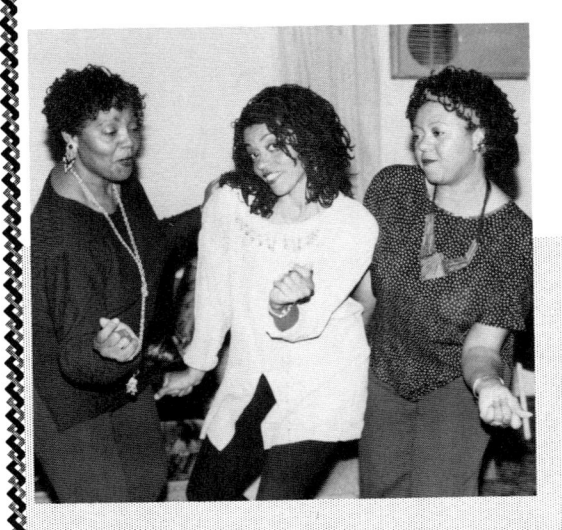

The Sisterlocks Sisters

I end this book with a tribute to sisterhood. My sisters, Celeste and Carol Jeanne, are my heart and my soul. Everything I know about sisterhood I learned from them. I see my image in their faces. When they laugh,

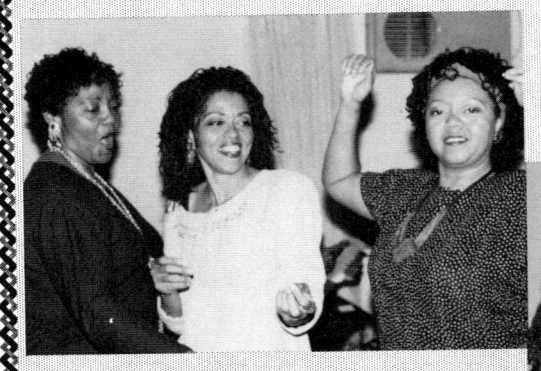

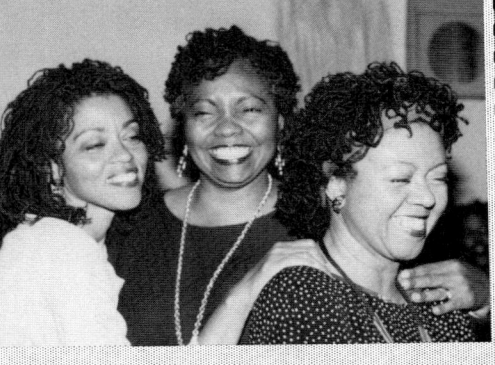

I laugh; when they cry, I cry. Nothing feels good for me if it is not also good for them.

The spirit of empathy we hold for each other was instilled in us by our mother, and is the basis of our business approach. Carol Jeanne has composed the following brief insight into how this empathy has played out for us, both as sisters and as business women.

THE SISTERLOCKS SISTERS
by Carol Jenkins

There is a saying that goes, "It's not where you start, it's where you finish." This saying seems a little inside out to me, because there's always something of where you started in where you finish. If not, then maybe it's because you have turned your back on an important part of who you really are!

It makes more sense to me to say, "It's where you start, AND where you finish." I'm sure that's because where my sisters and I started out has made all the difference in our lives. JoAnne has already described some of the experiences which helped to bring her to this stage with Sisterlocks. I'd like to add that our outlook, and much of our basic business philosophy, stems from being sisters, and more importantly, from the relationship we had with our mother.

Celeste and JoAnne are a year apart, and I came about 3 years later. The three of us could fill a room with our thick hair when it was freshly washed. It's no wonder my mother got a little

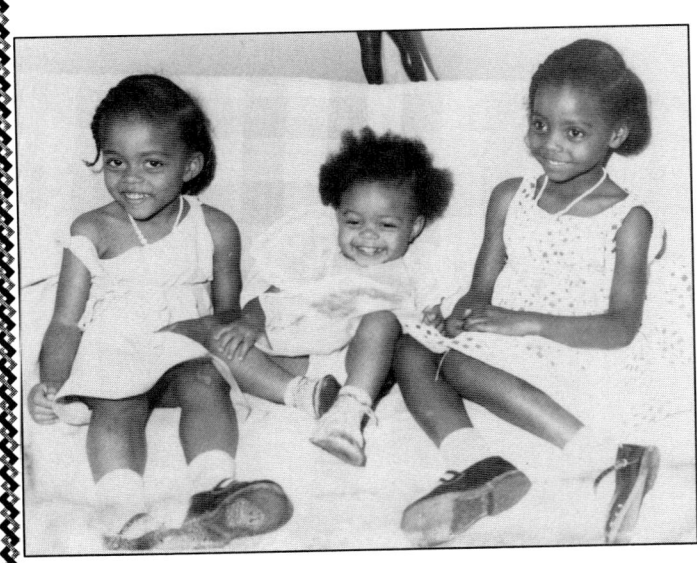

JoAnne, Carol Jeanne, Celeste

evil from time to time trying to yank that comb through it! Despite this, my most vivid impression is of how she taught us to be each other's best friend. "You've got the world to fight!" she would intone, adding in no uncertain terms that she would not stand for us fighting each other. She meant it too! In fact, she would spank all of us if she ever found us going at it. The imprint was made very early that we were in this thing together. We learned not to confuse our petty squabbles with the real life-battles that were waiting for us once we left the safety of home. We needed to stick together or we all might fall.

Now, I don't want you thinking that this kind of upbringing stifled our independence. I remember something that happened during the early 60's when Mom took us to buy some shoes. She needed to buy the sturdiest, but cheapest shoes she could find. Celeste and I got something pretty close to what we wanted, but for some reason, the ones she came up with for JoAnne were a horribly ugly pair of thick "crepe-soled" monstrosities. Celeste and I stood by helplessly aghast! These were "Old Lady" shoes! I mean, these things were nasty. Our friends were going to "cap" on JoAnne for years to come. Believe me, no kid would have willingly worn these shoes, and to her credit, neither did JoAnne.

The problem came when she said so to our mother. This was before kids told their parents what to do and, as you might expect, Mom didn't take that news too well. In fact, she was so amazed at my sister's impertinence that she couldn't contain herself. "This child must be outta her mind; She MUST be crazy!", she blared, or words to that affect. My fear for

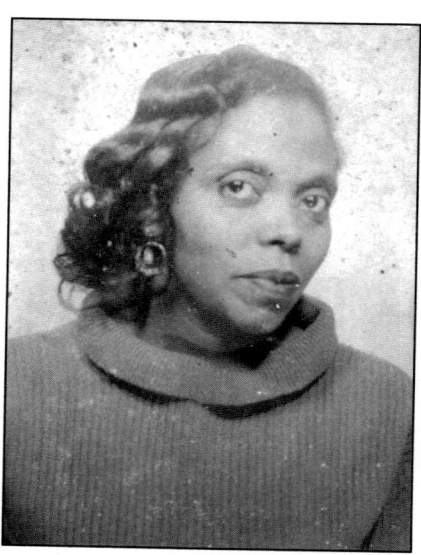

Dora Lee Smith Jenkins

my personal safety was eclipsed only by my fear that I was about to be minus one sister, just when I was starting to like her.

Not that Mom was abusive or such a strict disciplinarian, but there were certain things that any self-respecting, post World War II mom could not stand for, and SASS was one of them. All the while though, the three of us were picking up a heavy dose of sass through Mom's own example! We seem to have inherited some of Mom's contrariness too, but I think JoAnne got the largest dose. I know that both traits have been great assets to her in trying to develop the Sisterlocks concept.

Our oldest sister, Celeste, can be just plain stubborn sometimes. Unlike mom though, It's a quiet stubbornness - a sense of determination really - that's enveloped in a sweetness and vulnerability so seductive, I've never seen anyone, no matter how abrasive they might be, who could stand up to it. I think she got this quality from being the primary beneficiary of Mom's steadfast nurturing. They were the best of friends, even when we were young girls. Later, it was not uncommon for JoAnne and I to stumble out of bed at 9AM on Saturday, only to find Celeste and Mom, at the kitchen table since 6:30 or so, drinking coffee, eating boiled eggs, and figuring out life.

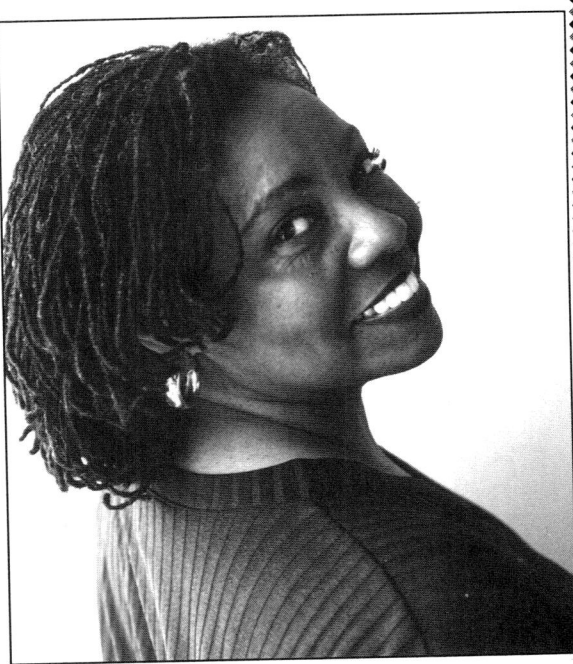

Celeste

Celeste is rock-solid, morally, spiritually, emotionally, and she brings that nurturing quality she learned from mom into everything she does. For sure, being a single mom placed financial stress on her, but she was completely in her element sharing and teaching love to her own children. Today she's a Certified Sisterlocks Consultant and Trainer, and her customers simply adore her. They come from far and wide. Some say that her hair care is like the laying on of hands. I think this is because she treats them all like sisters (and brothers) in the way we learned from our mother. Her standards for technical proficiency and customer satisfaction, are the ones we set forth as we train others in the Sisterlocks system.

As for me, well, JoAnne uses me as a sounding board. I guess this is because I picked up on mom's tendency to call things exactly like she saw them. (I was the baby girl, and could get away with this!) JoAnne relies on me to tell her when the emperor is not wearing any clothes. She also says she likes the way I help distill her sometimes obscure concepts down to "tasty little droplets that everyone and anyone can appreciate." I like things clear and uncomplicated. This is where the beauty of the Sisterlocks business lies, in my opinion.

Carol Jeanne

My sisters and I often jokingly say that if you

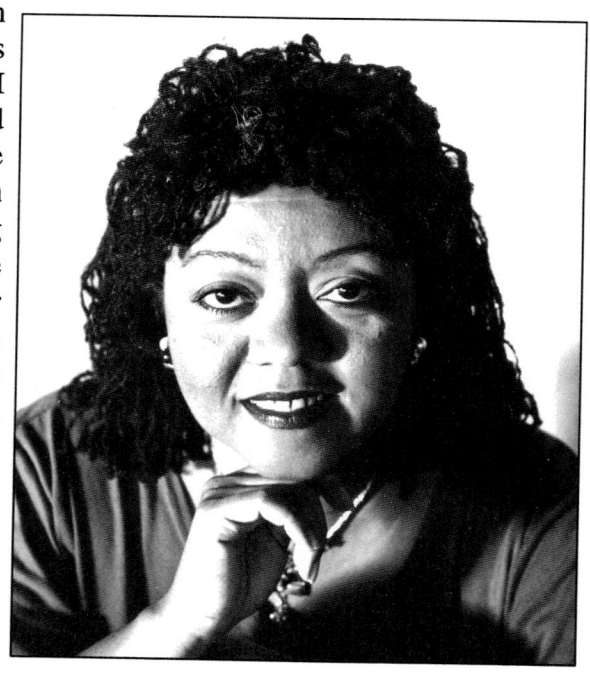

put the 3 of us together, we'd make up one hell of a good woman! As far as running the Sisterlocks business goes, I think this is true. We compliment each other amazingly well. JoAnne is the "head." She provides the vision, learning and technical insight that makes the system work. I guess I'm the "heart." JoAnne tells me she can read the pulse of African American sisterhood through my reactions to things. Also, having heart takes the drudgery out of the important, but more mundane daily tasks I have to perform to keep our business going. Celeste is definitely the "soul" of our enterprise. Through the disappointments and frustrations, she is our constant reminder of why we are doing this in the first place. She keeps our inspiration alive.

Lest you think my goal here is just to paint a family portrait, let me say that Sisterlocks is a kind of experiment in business development modeled on family and community dynamics. It's largely a learn-as-you-go enterprise. Oh, we've consulted with marketing specialists, and they have been helpful in many areas, but certain of our specific challenges have stumped them too. "How do you make a business fit with a characteristically black female approach to life?" "How do you transfer the principles of communication and exchange supportive of black family relationships, from that environment into the business realm?" Many of the traditional marketing techniques we looked at reminded us of the traditional hair techniques we have in our society. That is to say, they did not seem well suited to **our** culturally specific needs.

If we look at both small business and corporate models for doing business in America, we see they're built on assumptions that don't necessarily fit with the ways our people interact with each other in communities. Though none of us knew much about business starting out, we saw this, and it troubled us as we sat around the kitchen table trying to understand how to move our concepts and dreams forward. OUR bottom line is that we can't exactly "sell" our service at all, because so many of our women, though they may <u>need</u> it, may also see what we do as scary or threatening. A lot of what we must do is educate. We don't sell so much as open a door and extend an invitation. We have to create an environment where sisters want to join in with what we do. We must create that opportunity so they know they can come our way when they are ready. When they reach a level of acceptance where they can make that life change, they make a <u>commitment</u>, more than a purchase.

We don't do hype or high pressure sales. We're not creating a need in order to fill it. Our belief is that we can make a successful business that is consistent with the impulses of our culture - and that of black women especially - where giving is receiving.

Our business is simply based on the principles of good sisterhood as we learned these from our mother: Nurturing; mutual support and protection; long-term commitment to each other; and the conviction that we are dealing with something that is genuine, that is real, and that is OURS.

APPENDIX

172   That Hair Thing

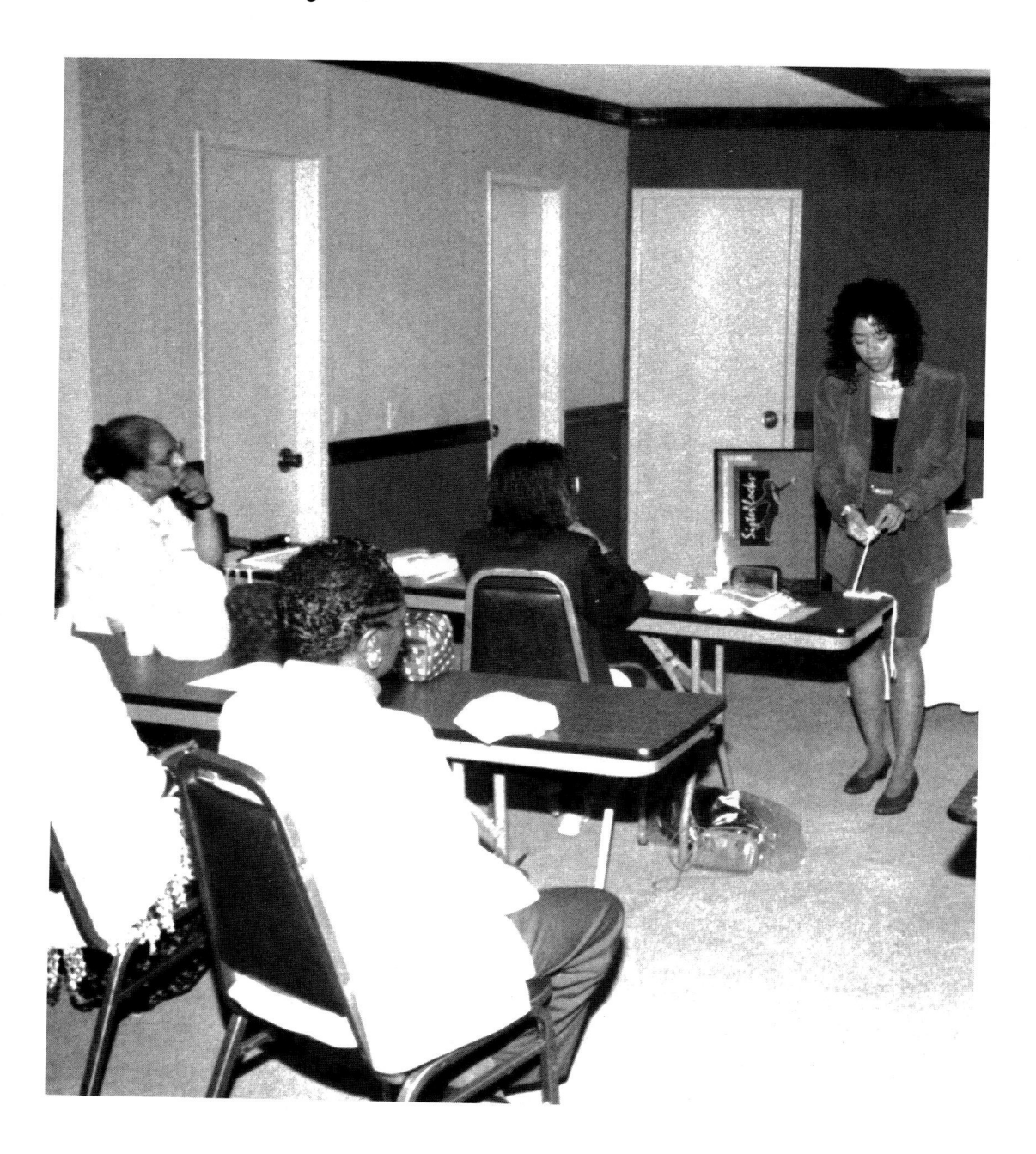

How To Find A Certified Sisterlocks Consultant:

The Certified Sisterlocks Consultant has completed a process that assures they have an acceptable level of proficiency in our system. They have had approximately 16 hours of course work and hands-on practice under the supervision of a Certified Training Associate. Following their training, Sisterlocks has tested their ability to perform our system on 3 clients independently.

Step 1
Phone the home office to find out if there is a Certified Consultant in your immediate area.

The home office keeps a registry of all of its Certified Consultants in good standing. Someone from our office will give you one or more names to contact, and unless you indicate otherwise, we will forward your information on to our Consultant(s) so they might contact you directly.

Step 2
(If there is no Certified Consultant in your area:)

Since Sisterlocks certification requires demonstration of customer satisfaction over time, there may be a trainee in your area who is an excellent technician, but who simply has not fully completed the certification process. The home office will also refer these people **as trainees**.

Step 3
(If there is no Consultant or trainee in your area:)

Hair care practitioners are business people who need to be sure they will have an adequate customer base before they learn a new technique. If you and others you know want Sisterlocks, find a reliable individual and encourage them to become trained in the system. Often, interested clients will actually "sponsor" someone to take the training, in exchange for getting their hair done. This creates a win/win situation for the business person and the client.

Sisterlocks trains individuals regardless of their previous training in cosmetology, braiding or hair locking.

What To Expect From A Certified Sisterlocks Consultant:

**Your Certified Consultant offers Sisterlocks as a package of 3 visits.
1) Before actually doing your hair, (s)he will do a thorough consultation, complete with sample locks being placed in your hair.
2) The second visit is your locking session. When you get your locks done, you will be given an official Customer Starter Kit, including the proper "Getting Started" shampoo, Washing Bands, and Tip Sheets to remind you about proper care.
3) Your Consultant will also do a follow-up visit with you after your hair is locked, to be sure your locks are behaving properly.**

Consultants are able to offer you the standard Sisterlocks locking services. The price for Sisterlocks is a package price, and is set by individual consultants.

Some Consultants are also cosmetologists and can offer you a range of other services like cutting, dying, scalp treatments, etc. Many of our Consultants who are not cosmetologists, can refer you to someone else for these services. The Sisterlocks home office is available to advise cosmetologists and others in our recommended shampooing, dying and trimming techniques for Sisterlocks.

Consultants are trained to work with the long term health of your natural hair in mind. They have access to a network of individuals with the resourses to advise them on every aspect of the Sisterlocks. Beyond this, it is important that you choose a Consultant you trust, and one with whom you can develop an open, honest relationship. This is the best guarantee of your long term satisfaction.

Sisterlocks : (619) 560-5116

How To Become Trained in the Sisterlocks System:

Our training system is designed to maximize the reliability of Sisterlocks services wherever they are offered.

Make sure you are trained by a Certified Training Associate. CTAs anywhere in the U.S. offer our standard curriculum:
BASIC (Classes 1-6) approx. 8hrs.
ADVANCED (Classes 7-9 plus marketing tips and hands-on) approx. 8-hrs.

Step 1
Enroll in the standardized training program.

Courses are offered at the home office in San Diego, or from our Certified Training Associates in several regions around the country. Our video assisted training approach is fully trademarked. Only CTAs are authorized to use these materials. These individuals have been trained in how to teach our standard methods.
Training consists of 9 classes covering the following areas:

Day 1: classes 1 - 6
1) The Characteristics of Naturally Textured Hair, 2) Sisterlocks Locking Patterns; 3) Parting, Sectioning and Lock Sizes; 4) Finger Positions and Tool Applications; 5) The Hair's Natural Interlocking Process; 6) Shampooing Techniques.

Day 2: classes 7 - 9
7) Re-Tightening and Remedy Techniques; 8) Troubleshooting and Fixing Things; 9) The Sisterlocks Consultation.

Day 2 of the training program also includes a discussion of marketing techniques for Sisterlocks, and helps trainees understand their business relationship with our trademarked company.

Step 2
Complete the certification requirements.

After completing all course work, trainees are eligible for our private certification. They must do 3 customers independently, and submit all appropriate paperwork including photos. Following an approval process from the home office, trainees will become Certified as Sisterlocks Consultants.

Certified Consultants become part of a national registry of properly trained practitioners of the Sisterlocks system, committed to delivering brand name quality services to their customers. This registry is reviewed and updated quarterly. Certified Consultants in good standing receive referrals from the home office, special pricing and distributor rights on products and accessories, and access to advertising and promotional opportunities. They also receive a quarterly newsletter that keeps them updated on relevant issues and provides tips and information to improve and refine their techniques. The home office is available to them at any time for troubleshooting or problem solving relative to the Sisterlocks system.

Step 3
Become a Certified Training Associate.

Once Consultants have acquired enough confidence and skill in working with their Sisterlocks customer base, they may take our course to become a Certified Training Associate. The training curriculum includes one full day of classes on how to teach our standardized curriculum, and a full day of supervised teaching practice.

CTAs are then licensed to offer the standardized Sisterlocks training curriculum in their own cities and regions. These are the same as those offered by the home office. Individuals trained by them are also eligible for Certification as Consultants through the home office.

...

Regulations for practicing natural hair care as a business vary from state to state. For ongoing information and guidelines in these matters, we recommend our Consultants become members of the American Hairbraiders and Natural Haircare Association (AHNHA) (202) 723-5495

For Information on Regional Training Schedules Call or Write:

Sisterlocks

5663 Balboa Ave. #355
San Diego, Ca 92111
(619) 687-7853
(recorded message)

ORDER FORM

ITEM QUAN. TOTAL

That Hair Thing (book)
(Share the Sisterlocks gift with family and friends!) $19.95ea.

"That Hair Thing" (video tape-18 min.)
(A moving discussion by Dr. Cornwell on how our women's hair issues affect our lives.) $14.95ea.

"Come Home To Sisterlocks" (video - 18min.)
(Many Sisterlocks 'looks'; Individuals speak of styling, friends' reactions and more! Plus, Dr. Cornwell walks you through the care routine.) $14.95ea.

Logo T-Shirt
Black with white logo. XL only. ($17.50)

Sisterlocks Product Kit ($18.95)
8oz. Spray Shampoo / 8oz. Moisture Treat. / 16oz. Reconstruct/Cond.
Indicate hair type: Wavy ___ Average ___ Tight Texture ___

Shipping and Handling:
First book/video/T-Shirt - $3.50
Additional books/videos/T-Shirts - $1.00ea.

SUB-TOTAL _____
ADD S & H _____
GRAND TOTAL _____

Please send me information on:
Sisterlocks training classes in my region. ☐   A Certified Consultant in my area ☐

Name: _____

Address: _____
_____
_____

SEND CHECK OR MONEY ORDER TO:

Sisterlocks

**5663 Balboa Avenue #355
San Diego, CA 92111**

(For Check Orders - allow 3-4wk delivery)

CALL TO PLACE YOUR CREDIT CARD ORDER TODAY! (619) 560-5116

ORDER FORM

ITEM	QUAN.	TOTAL
That Hair Thing (book) (Share the Sisterlocks gift with family and friends!) $19.95ea.	_____	_____
"That Hair Thing" (video tape-18 min.) (A moving discussion by Dr. Cornwell on how our women's hair issues affect our lives.) $14.95ea.	_____	_____
"Come Home To Sisterlocks" (video - 18min.) (Many Sisterlocks 'looks'; Individuals speak of styling, friends' reactions and more! Plus, Dr. Cornwell walks you through the care routine.) $14.95ea.	_____	_____
Logo T-Shirt Black with white logo. XL only. ($17.50)	_____	_____
Sisterlocks Product Kit ($18.95) 8oz. Spray Shampoo / 8oz. Moisture Treat. / 16oz. Reconstruct/Cond. Indicate hair type: Wavy ___ Average ___ Tight Texture ___	_____	_____

SUB-TOTAL _____

ADD S & H _____

GRAND TOTAL _____

Shipping and Handling:
First book/video/T-Shirt - $3.50
Additional books/videos/T-Shirts - $1.00ea.

Please send me information on:
Training classes in my region. ☐   A Certified Consultant in my area ☐

Name: _____

Address: _____

_____

_____

SEND CHECK OR MONEY ORDER TO:

Sisterlocks

5663 Balboa Avenue #355
San Diego, CA 92111

(For Check Orders - allow 3-4 wk delivery)

CALL TO PLACE YOUR CREDIT CARD ORDER TODAY! (619) 560-5116